Client Profile

Adul
and th   rly

Client Profiles in Nursing

Adult
and the Elderly

Edited by

P Simpson MSc DipEd Cert Ed DN (Lond) RCNT RN

School of Health Studies
University of Portsmouth
Portsmouth

T Okubadejo MSc BSc (Hons) PGCEA RN RM PGDipHV

Southampton Community
NHS Trust
Southampton

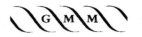

© 2001

Greenwich Medical Media Limited
137 Euston Road
London
NW1 2AA

ISBN 1 84110 000 5

First published 2001

Visit our website at:
www.greenwich-medical.co.uk

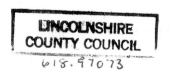
Distributed worldwide by Plymbridge Distributors Ltd

Typeset by Phoenix Photosetting, Chatham
Printed in Ashford Colour Press Ltd, Hants

Contents

Client profiles in nursing: adults & the elderly

Client profiles in nursing: adults & the elderly

This series of learning aids has been designed for use by pre-registration student nurses, their assessors, nurse educationalists and healthcare support workers undertaking NVQ level 3. Their purpose is to simulate as far as possible in writing, the kinds of complex human situations which registered and unregistered practitioners are likely to encounter in the course of their work and which will influence assessment and decision making in terms of nursing management.

Each volume may be used for revision purposes, to generate ideas about producing case profiles or as a basis for compiling question for use with learners.

The authors are all highly experienced registered nurses, who have compiled the profiles utilising their areas of specialist knowledge and professional experience. 'Truth', as the saying goes, 'is stranger than fiction' and we hope that the cases reflect this perversity, which most clinical nurses will recognise at once to be the case!

This volume has been written with the nursing of adults in mind and there has been a deliberate attempt to present a balanced range of ages, ethnic backgrounds, gender, social circumstances, acute and chronic conditions and healthcare settings (community and hospital) to stimulate readers' thinking and to focus thought away from purely pathological matters. The editors have attempted to reflect the reality of the National Health Service, which is that the majority of nursing occurs with chronic conditions and in primary care or community settings. Health promotion is also emphasised, reflecting contemporary health policy.

The questions posed range from those which are short and descriptive, based on anatomy and physiology, to very complex management questions. The latter will require some time to identify the main issues and subsequently to prioritise these.

Each case profile consists of a scenario, questions and model answers, a reference list and suggestions for further reading.

How to use this book for revision

It is suggested that readers will need to have the following to hand: a nursing or medical dictionary, a pharmacology textbook and an anatomy and physiology textbook in order to maximise their use of time.

The index outlines the main topic areas for each case profile. It is assumed that the reader who wishes to use this volume for revision purposes will have learned the relevant topic area prior to answering the questions!

Each scenario should be read through carefully, with notes made of the main points. The questions should then be read. The clockface logo by each question will give you an estimate of the timescale involved for thinking about and planning your answer. Whenever you are ready, turn over the page to view the answers. You may wish to develop your answers by further reading.

- Questions may be dealt with one at a time or in a block
- Further volumes will deal with paediatric nursing, and more care of the adult patient
- If you would like to submit profiles for inclusion in future volumes in this series, we would be delighted to hear from you.

The editors and authors very much hope that readers will enjoy working with this book, since we believe that learning is much easier where the mind is having fun! Happy learning!

Tinuade Okubadejo
February, 2001

Chris Buswell
Staff Nurse/Freelance Nurse Writer
Grove Court Residential/Nursing Home
Elizabeth Finn Trust
Suffolk, UK

Debra Elliott, MSc, BSc (Hons) RGN, Cert HE Cert Ed (FE) RNT
Senior Nurse
Medical Division
Portsmouth Hospitals NHS Trust

Bernard Mark Garrett, BSc (Hons), PGCE, RGN, RNT
Principal Lecturer
School of Health Care
Oxford Brookes University
Oxford

Anthony J Holland, BSc (Hons), RN, Dip HE (NS), EMT
Occupational Health Nurse Industry
Portsmouth

Barbara Marjoram, TD, MA, RN, CertED
Deputy Head of Pre Registration Education
School of Nursing and Midwifery
University of Southampton

Vivienne Mathews, RGN RNT CertEd
School of Health Studies
Queen Alexandra Hospital
Portsmouth

Tinuade Okubadejo, MSc, BSc, RN, RM, RHV, PGCEA
Senior Lecturer
Southampton Community NHS Trust
Southampton

Chris Pearce, RN, BSc, MA, PGCEA
Senior Lecturer
South Bank University

Carmel Sheppard, RGN, BSc (Hons), MSc, Dip Counselling
Breast Care Nurse Specialist
Portsmouth Hospitals NHS Trust

Penelope Simpson, MSc DipEd Cert Ed DN (Lond) RCNT RN
School of Health Studies
Queen Alexandra Hospital
Portsmouth

Abdominoperineal resection

Vivienne Mathews

Robin Fraser is 65 years of age and has just retired from work as a bus driver. He is married to Gwen, who is 58 years old and works for the Halifax Building Society as a teller. They have three children, aged 30, 27 and 24 years. Both Rob (as he likes to be called) and Gwen enjoy a game of cards in their local community centre and, as they are keen gardeners, they belong to the local allotment society, where Gwen has taken on the role of secretary. Rob also plays skittles for the British Legion team.

Rob and Gwen were looking forward to their youngest child finally leaving home and going to university, after an anxious time when he travelled, backpacking, round the world. They had planned a Mediterranean cruise, but through family circumstances and Rob's ill health, it had to be abandoned.

Three months before his hospital admission, Rob visited his general practitioner (GP) with a 2-month history of a constant desire to have his bowels open and the frequent passage of small, liquid stools. Otherwise, he felt fit and well, with no other symptoms.

A sigmoidoscopy was performed and a large mass was found in his rectum. Biopsy results showed a large tumour in the rectum, near the anal margin, which proved to be malignant, but localised to the bowel. A barium enema confirmed the presence and extent of the tumour. A surgical admission was planned for an abdominoperineal resection and formation of colostomy.

Question one: Discuss the pathology of rectal carcinoma, the rate of growth and spread, and the treatment.

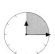

15 minutes

Question two: What problems of body image and lifestyle are likely to be encountered by Rob and Gwen?

10 minutes

Question three: Describe a teaching programme for Rob to enable him to cope with his new stoma.

15 minutes

Time allowance: **40 minutes**

Answer to question one:
Discuss the pathology of rectal carcinoma, the rate of growth and spread, and the treatment.

The commonest malignant tumour of the rectum is usually carcinoma. This condition affects men and women of all ages equally, with the highest incidence occurring in the elderly population (Hogstel, 1992). It has been suggested that diet, especially one high in fat with a low residue and bulk, may be a cause of colonic cancer, but the exact cause is as yet unknown (Hogstel, 1992).

Cancer is the growth of new cells in the mucous membrane of the rectum or of malignant changes in existing papilloma and/or glands of the rectum (adenoma). Initially, the growth spreads to local areas; it is only later that it invades the deeper layers of tissue around the perimeter of the bowel. Cancer can also spread via the lymphatic system, so that lymph glands immediately adjacent to the rectum will be involved. Eventually it will spread to those of the large bowel mesentery and the lymph glands around the heart. Cancer cells are also spread via the bloodstream, finally arriving in the liver, lungs and bones (Sands & Dennison, 1995).

It is unfortunate that the first symptom to be noticed is usually a blob of bright red blood, which is often mistaken for 'piles' and so is ignored. There will be sensations of having a full rectum, of wanting to defecate frequently and of pain. If a diagnosis can be made before these symptoms appear then surgical treatment is very successful, but if the condition is not treated there will be rectal obstruction, with lower abdominal pain, accompanied by alternating bouts of diarrhoea and constipation.

Diagnosis is confirmed by the following tests:

- Digital examination
- Sigmoidoscopy
- Barium enema
- Biopsy
- Samples sent for histological examination.

Cancer in the lower part of the rectum is often very close to the anal sphincter. If this is the case, the rectum, with its mesentery, and the anus are surgically removed, while the remaining bowel is brought out through the abdominal wall to form a colostomy. This operation is performed by two surgeons, one working from the inside of the abdomen, and the other working from the perineum (Parboteeah, 1998).

Answer to question two:
What problems of body image and lifestyle are likely to be encountered by Rob and Gwen?

Kelly (1994) states that patients who have operations that result in the formation of a stoma often have second thoughts about the operation and their ability to cope. If there is to be a long-term change in the patient's concept of self,
the reality of the situation has to be accepted and acknowledged before the
operation can take place.

Rob may have anxieties about the effect a colostomy would have on his family and upon himself. He may be unsure about the implications of having a
colostomy. He may not be able to discuss his fears with his wife or a nurse
whom he perceives to be younger than his grand-daughter. Kelly (1994) also
suggests that in order for a patient to master use of a stoma they have to be in
control of it, not vice versa.

Postoperatively, there may be difficulties in coming to terms with the
actuality of having a stoma. It could be that, although teaching has taken
place pre-operatively, the reality of having to empty and change a stoma
appliance may not have sunk in. Elcoat (1986) recognised this as suppression,
when a patient is reluctant or suppresses the presence of the stoma, uncon-
sciously excluding information so that they are unable to learn about stoma
care.

Rob may feel embarrassed by the smell emanating from the stoma; the sight
of it may make him feel 'dirty' or nauseated. He will not be able to control his
urge to defecate and this fact, according to Tschudin (1988), will have a powerful impact on Rob's self-worth and his consequent loss of dignity as he strug-
gles to overcome feelings of being unclean and socially unacceptable.

Kelly & Henry (1993) state that if identified issues have not been resolved
and worked through in the first postoperative week, there will be profound
effects on the subsequent quality of life. Time and space will be needed to work
out problems and air negative feelings.

Both Borwell (1997) and MacArthur (1996) state that their colostomy patients
often have worries about sexual matters. According to Borwell (1997), sexuality
is an area of care that is often seen as the nurse's responsibility, but which some
nurses find stressful, especially if the patient, like Rob, is unable to talk about it.
He was sexually active before his operation and it may be 2–3 months before
sexual intercourse can be resumed. There is a possibility that sexual activity will
be hindered owing to loss of libido or difficulty with ejaculation; sexual counselling should be offered prior to the operation (Parboteeah, 1998). There may
be some sense of revulsion with regard to the stoma, or there may be fear that
pain or damage to the stoma may occur during sexual activity; these issues will
have to be addressed.

Tschudin (1988) suggested that a general enquiry along the lines of 'How do
you feel your surgery will affect your partner?' may elicit a response that will
reveal how both Gwen and Rob feel about the stoma. In conversation with them
both, try to find out what has been said to family and friends, as it may be possible that cancer and surgery have been mentioned, but not information about
the stoma. Kelly (1994) identifies this lack of information giving on the part of

the patient as a potential problem and suggests that a rehearsal may make the situation more palatable for the future.

It is important that nurses are aware of their own limitations in this field and can find someone who will deal with the issue in an appropriate way, as the need for accurate, relevant information will not have been met (MacArthur, 1996).

Answer to question three:
Describe a teaching programme for Rob to enable him to cope with his new stoma.

A stoma nurse specialist should be involved with Rob and Gwen both pre-operatively and post-operatively, to help with siting the stoma, to educate and guide the patient toward learning new skills in dealing with the appliance, and to facilitate the acceptance of a changed body image.

One of the priorities of care will be teaching Rob the technique of changing the stoma appliance.

The following items and information are needed for education and training:

- A bathroom that is warm, private and comfortable
- Available hot water for cleansing
- A mirror to check the correct position of the appliance
- Diagrams of stoma function and relevant anatomy and physiology
- An explanation and practise on how to remove the appliance
- A demonstration of the site, colour and size of the stoma
- An explanation of the importance of good skin care
- A discussion of the safe disposal of soiled appliances
- An explanation of the procedures and then an observation of the patient doing them for himself in safe, non-judgemental circumstances
- Time to practice should be allowed so that the task can be accomplished with ease and dexterity.

(Adapted from Thompson, 1998)

The nurse's role, initially, will be to guide and direct proceedings, giving small amounts of information as needed, for example the choice of appliances available to Rob, methods of cleaning and safe application of each appliance.

If both Gwen and Rob agree, Gwen should be invited to attend these training sessions so that she can take over the care of the stoma if it ever becomes necessary.

Stress and anxiety can be avoided if communication between nurses, stoma therapists and patients is considered of paramount importance. Then, with the skills and knowledge of how to manage his stoma, Rob will achieve acceptance and adaptation will surely follow.

References

Borwell, B. (1997). The psychosexual needs of the stoma patient. Professional Nurse 12(4): 250–255.

Elcoat, C. (1986). Stoma Care Nursing. Sussex: Balliere Tindall.

Hogstel, M. O. (1992). Clinical Manual of Gerontological Nursing. St Louis: Mosby Yearbook.

Kelly, M., Henry, T. (1993). Open discussion can lead to acceptance: the psychological effects of stoma surgery. Professional Nurse 9(2): 101–110.

Kelly, M. (1994). Mind and body. Nursing Times 90(42): 48–51.

MacArthur, A. (1996). Sexuality and the stoma: helping patients to cope. Nursing Times 92(39): 34–35.

Parboteeah, S. (1998). Gastrointestinal surgery. In: Simpson, P. M. (Ed.) Introduction to Surgical Nursing. London: Arnold.

Sands, J. K., Dennison, E. (1995). Clinical Manual of Medical-Surgical Nursing. St Louis: Mosby Yearbook.

Thomson, I. (1998). Teaching skills to cope with a stoma. Nursing Times 94(4): 55–56.

Tschudin, V. (1988). Nursing the Patient with Cancer. Cambridge: Prentice Hall.

Further reading

Price, B. (1990). Body image – nursing concepts and care. Cambridge: Prentice Hall.

Abuse: non-accidental injury

Vivienne Mathews

> Harold Winterstoke is a 71-year-old widower, who lives with his daughter, Sally, son-in-law, Colin, and their three children. They occupy a semi-detached house in the middle of a large council housing estate.
>
> Harold is thin, frail and underweight for his 1.77 m (5′ 10″) frame. He is a retired bus driver, who gave up his council flat when he fell and sustained a fractured femur. This resulted in an arthrodesis. Since his hospitalisation, he has not regained his former level of independence, and has become unsteady on his feet and more and more forgetful.
>
> Colin, his son-in-law, offered the smallest bedroom in the house to Harold, moving his three children together into one bedroom. Harold was to pay for his keep and give his personal effects (TV, microwave oven, dining table and chairs, collection of musical instruments and large Welsh dresser) to his daughter. This arrangement appeared to suit them all at first, as extra money coming into the house eased some of their financial problems and provided holidays for them all.
>
> Sadly, the family situation deteriorated as Harold became more and more forgetful and he developed Alzheimer's disease. His negative behaviour and anti-social habits of faecal soiling and eating his food noisily, coupled with his constant calling out for his dead wife, have worsened relationships within the family.
>
> Harold was admitted to the Accident & Emergency (A & E) department with severe bruising to his right shoulder and arm, a broken nose and split frenulum. His right eye was discoloured and extremely swollen. Colin stated that Harold had fallen down the stairs during the night.

Question one: Outline prevalence, definitions and types of abuse that may be suffered by elderly people.

15 minutes

Question two: What factors in Mr Winterstoke's living arrangements have led to his being physically abused?

10 minutes

Question three: What are the factors that indicate that a non-accidental injury has occurred (Fig. 1)?

10 minutes

Time allowance: **35 minutes**

Answer to question one:
Outline prevalence, definitions and types of abuse that may be suffered by elderly people.

It has been estimated that 32 in every 1000 people over the age of 60 are victims of abuse of some sort; that is 32% of the total population in the UK (Baumhover & Beall, 1996). Pritchard (1998) states that one-third of all victims of abuse are male and that the age of the majority of victims is not over 80, but mostly between 60 and 80 years old.

Abuse of the elderly person has been defined as being either physical, sexual, psychological or financial. It may be intentional, unintentional or the result of neglect. It causes harm to the elderly person, either temporarily or over a period of time (Social Services Inspectorate, 1992).

Elder abuse is the mistreatment of an older person that results in suffering and distress (Royal College of Nursing, 1996). These guidelines go on to say that abuse can be passive as well as active, and that it occurs frequently as a result of carers lacking the knowledge of how to respond to an elderly person's needs, or because they are overburdened and torn by conflicting demands, lacking in strength of will to continue with an intolerable situation.

Abuse, then, can be defined in various ways, as can the types of abuse that are perpetrated on elderly people:

1. *Physical abuse*: the infliction of harm
   - Abrasions and lacerations
   - Burns
   - Freezing
   - Fractures and sprains
   - Dehydration
   - Inappropriate clothing
   - Untreated medical problems
   - Punching
   - Restraint
   - Over medication
   - Bondage
   - Malnutrition
   - Poor hygiene
   - Over-sedation
   - Rough handling.

   (Adapted from Kingston & Penhale, 1995)

2. *Psychological abuse*: the infliction of mental anguish
   - Threats: verbal assault
   - Ignoring
   - Patronising
   - Name calling
   - Offensive language
   - Taking revenge
   - Ridiculing
   - Bullying

- Witholding affection
- Humiliation
- Harassment (by local children)
- Removal of dignity and privacy
- Removal of decision making.

(Action on Elder Abuse, 1995)

3. *Material abuse*: illegal or improper exploitation of funds and/or resources
   - Theft
   - Misuse of money or property
   - Fraud
   - Exploitation
   - Failure to meet legal obligations
   - Denial of pension rights.

4. *Sexual abuse*: coercing or forcing an elderly person to take part in any sexual activity without consent
   - Rape
   - Forcing elderly people to look at pornographic or sexually explicit material
   - Involvement in conversations that have sexual connotations or innuendo
   - 'Dirty' joke telling
   - Inappropriate touching or fondling.

5. *Neglect*: the wilful or non-wilful failure by care giver to fulfil their caretaking obligations or duties (Penhale, 1995)
   - Witholding food, drink, warmth, comfort or medication
   - Smelling of urine or faeces
   - Restricting mobility by:
     a) Being hemmed in or trapped in a chair
     b) Lack of aids. 'I can't let her have a frame, she'll fall and hurt herself.'
     c) Lack of space or knowledge
   - Isolation
   - Denial of social contact
   - When essential needs are not met, e.g. hygiene
   - Lack of stimulation
   - Undermining personal beliefs.

(Adapted from Carter, 1999)

6. *Institutional abuse*: abuse of power
   - Compulsory bath/shower/strip wash
   - Compulsory bowel care
   - Misuse of medication
   - Dressing inappropriately
   - Ridiculing
   - 'Telling off' as a child
   - Ignoring requests
   - Restraint
   - Taking away treasured possessions
   - Putting to bed too early.

Answer to question two:
What factors in Mr Winterstoke's living arrangements have led to his being physically abused?

There are many theories about why elderly people become the victims of abuse:

- Dependent impairment theories
- Stressed care giver theory
- Family violence set of learned behaviours
- Role reversal theory
- Pathological personality theory.

(Bennett, 1990)

It is possible that the first theory mentioned above, or a combination of several of them, apply to Mr Winterstoke and his family.

When a residence is shared with the principle carer, the elderly person is likely to be at risk of abuse (Social Services Inspectorate, 1992). Harold is dependent on his family, particularly his daughter, for all his daily needs. This constitutes a reversal of roles, from adult to that of child, which may not have been forseen, or welcomed, by the family members. As his condition deteriorates, his daughter, Sally, has to spend more and more time caring for her father, to the detriment of her other duties towards her husband, her sons and herself. Colin, in his turn, is resentful of the time and energy she expends on her father and resorts to violence to ease his frustrations.

There is also the possibility of financial abuse within this family, as Harold is no longer capable of managing his own affairs.

What is clear is that Mr Winterstoke falls into many of the categories designated as the 'classic victim' of abuse.

The classic victim of abuse is:

- Physically frail
- Female
- Over 65 years of age
- Dependent on others for many activities of living
- Living with carers
- Being overweight (hard to lift)
- Lost communication skills
- Immobile
- Onset of dementia
- Incontinent
- Possessing negative personality traits, e.g. hitting out, biting, spitting, faecal art.

(Eastman, 1984)

Mr Winterstoke did not confide in A & E staff because of the need to maintain family loyalty and secrecy. He may well believe the family unit is private; a domain where intrusions are resented and strangers asking questions are not welcome.

Abuse always occurs without witnesses, so there may be an element of fear, shame or embarrassment involved. Retaliation may have occurred on previous occasions, or Mr Winterstoke may be thinking that it is 'God's will' or that he is being punished for past misdemeanours. Because of his increasing dementia he may be unable to articulate his situation, and may believe that the abuse will stop 'one day'. It could also be normal behaviour within this family (Staab & Hodges, 1996).

Client profiles in nursing: adults & the elderly

Answer to question three:
What are the factors that indicate a non-accidental injury has occurred (Fig. 2.1)?

Careful questioning may reveal that the three generational family live in cramped accommodation, with high levels of stress caused by the physical dependence of Mr Winterstoke. This, coupled with other factors mentioned below may have alerted the medical and nursing staff to the possibility of non-accidental injury:

- There may be conflicting explanations of the injury
- There may be discrepancies in the history given by Colin and Mr Winterstoke
- There may have been a long delay in reporting and treating injuries
- There may be evidence of multiple injuries in various stages of repair
- Denial from Harold that he is hurt may show that he is threatened and intimidated by Colin
- Harold may be over-anxious to please his son-in-law
- Harold may be passive, withdrawn and not show any interest in his care.

(Phillips, 1983)

Injuries:

- black eye right side
- fractured nose
- split frenulum
- bruising right shoulder
- bruising right arm

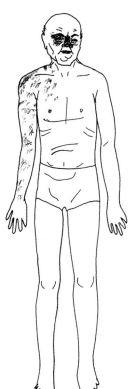

Suggestive signs:

- expressionless face
- dementia
- dysphasic
- dry tongue
- injury to ear, black eye
- bruised jaw
- unused hearing aid or glasses
- pinch marks
- urine rash
- kick marks on legs with other signs of non-accidental injury
- pressure sores

Diagnostic signs:

- finger and thumb marks over the shoulders
- multiple little bruises over the sternum/back
- cowering when approached
- isolated room
- poor conditions in comparison with rest of household
- old, inadequate clothing
- inadequate heating
- food in hair

Figure 2.1: Non-accidental injury.

Ostrow, C.L. (1997). The use of the Trendelenburg position by critical care nurses. American Journal of Critical Care 6(3): 172–176.

Smith, T. (1997). Renal Nursing. London: Baillière Tindall.

Taylor, C. Lillis, C., LeMone, P. (1997). Fundamentals of Nursing; the Art and Science of Nursing Care. Cheltenham: Stanley Thornes Ltd. (Lippincott).

Further reading

Solowij, N., Hall, W., Lee, N. (1992). Recreational MDMA use in Sydney: a profile of 'Ecstasy' users and their experiences with the drug. British Journal of Addiction 87(8): 1161–1172.

Walsh, M. (Ed) (1997). Watson's Clinical Nursing & Related Sciences, 5th Edn. London: Baillière Tindall.

Alcohol abuse

Vivienne Mathews

'My father-in-law is only 67 years old, but he looks 87. He is a widower who lives alone in a huge four bedroomed house that is far too big for him to manage. So he wanders around, using mainly the ground floor. You know, the kitchen, toilet and breakfast room where it appears that he sleeps.

He was referred to a private agency for a home help as he seemed unable to manage every day things like cooking, shopping, cleaning and his laundry. I thought his mind was going. Well, he hasn't been the same since he gave up work years ago. My wife, Eileen, used to visit him regularly. She changed his bed linen, did some shopping for him and took his washing home with her, but recently he has refused to let Eileen into the house. Left her standing on the doorstep, shouting at him through the letter box. He just ignored her. He lets me in, though.

The home help visited him, daily, for a while, to do housework and monitor the situation. She thinks he's got dementia as he can't remember much, but she does say he's 'spot on' where money is concerned. She also says he has some unusual habits. For example, he doesn't use the toilet properly and only eats bread and cheese! He also drinks a lot of sherry. She finds six or seven empty bottles each week. Where he gets it from, I don't know!

He won't let anyone in, now, except me and I found him walking around with no clothes on the other day. The house is filthy, the home help won't go in any more. She says its a health hazard. Cecil was referred to a community psychiatric nurse (CPN), who stated that he was not mentally ill, not sectionable and reported the situation to the GP, who refuses to visit until the house is cleaned, but Cecil won't let me do anything about it, only collect his pension.'

Question one: Do elderly people form a distinct group of alcohol abusers?

10 minutes

Question two: Discuss the effects of alcohol on an elderly person's body.

15 minutes

Question three: What treatment is available for Mr Ingram?

15 minutes

Time allowance: **40 minutes**

Client profiles in nursing: adults & the elderly

Answer to question one:
Do elderly people form a distinct group of alcohol abusers?

In the UK over 4000 deaths per year were attributed to alcohol compared with 1620 drug-related deaths (OPCS, 1993). Alcohol-related mortality has risen by one-third since 1984 and among people under the age of 45, the increase is even greater, yet alcohol consumption seems to be regarded with benign tolerance and is promoted as being 'cool' or 'sophisticated' (Insight, 1998).

Drinking that adversely affects physical health, behaviour, relationships and/or employment is considered heavy or problem drinking (Barbor, 1993).

It has been stated by Malcolm (1992) that as many as one elderly person in 10 has an alcohol-related problem. Many reasons for this are given. Leach (1999) states that the elderly, as a group, are bored and lonely; they need help to regain their former levels of self-esteem and become active again.

McCracken (1998) stresses that 80% of people over the age of 65 have at least one chronic illness, and that depression accompanying impaired health may cause elderly people to drink. Roberts (1988) has looked at patterns of drinking in elderly people and states that elderly people drink, on the whole, less than young people. She feels that many previously heavy drinkers would by now be dead from alcohol-related problems, and that elderly people are often on low incomes and cannot, literally, afford to drink. She also says that elderly people are aware of the risks associated with drinking, e.g. falls, and so control their intake accordingly.

It may be that elderly people are following the trend set by younger people and are drinking more. After all, there has been a fall in the relative cost of alcohol. It is easily available in all supermarkets and convenience stores. TV advertising presents alcohol as a homely, pleasurable pastime. Pubs are now friendly towards women and the blurring of sex roles has made drinking acceptable for women.

Malcolm (1992) claims that there are two types of elderly drinkers:

1. *Group one:*
   - Both sexes equally represented
   - Tend to be younger (60–75 years)
   - Heavy drinkers
   - Preoccupied by drink (where the next one is coming from!)
   - Suffer social consequences of drunkenness
   - Suffer withdrawal symptoms of: nausea ,sweating, panicking, epileptic fits, craving drink, trembling, lack of appetite, delirium tremens
   - May be evidence of alcohol-induced dementia
   - Brain damage, e.g. Korsakov's psychosis
   - Disordered liver functions
   - Pancreatitis
   - Peripheral neuropathy
   - Dies before reaching old age.

2. *Group two:*
   - Start to abuse alcohol late in life

- More women than men (5:1)
- Over 75 when drinking reaches problem status
- Take to drink to escape stress
- Distressed over bereavement, retirement, loneliness or poor health
- May be related to the onset of dementia
- Loss of inhibitions – removes social controls on behaviour
- Loss of judgement – makes matters worse
- Clinically depressed.

(Adapted from Malcolm, 1992)

It is clear that many elderly people drink alcohol, but that is no different from other groups of people who enjoy drinking as a pleasant, sociable behaviour. Each elderly person has a choice about how much to drink and when, so with education, information and encouragement support can be given when the problem of alcohol abuse is evident.

It would seem that Mr Ingram fits into both the groups of drinkers. He is from a younger age group, drinks heavily and has no social life. There may also be evidence of alcohol-induced dementia; equally he may be drinking to relieve the stress of his retirement and widower status. He is disinhibited and possibly clinically depressed.

Symptoms, such as malnutrition, confusion and self-neglect often disguise alcohol problems and are less likely to be identified by health care professionals (Leach, 1999).

Client profiles in nursing: adults & the elderly

Answer to question two:
Discuss the effects of alcohol on the elderly person's body.

Alcohol affects elderly people badly because:

- The elderly brain is increasingly vulnerable to alcohol; the tolerance to alcohol that regular drinkers develop is lost
- The elderly body has a greater proportion of fat to water, in consequence as alcohol dissolves in fluids, so blood alcohol levels are concentrated, having a deleterious effect on the brain and other organs
- Excessive intake of alcohol causes malnutrition. The metabolism of alcohol uses simple enzyme systems and if used in excess, for an appreciable length of time, the metabolic pathways used for more complex chemicals of a balanced diet and drugs become inactivated

  Elderly people may become malnourished for other reasons but, because of decreased energy levels, decreased repair and growth processes, do not need as many calories as younger people. Alcohol has no nutritional value at all. If alcohol replaces normal dietary elements, nutritional deficiencies will develop. If alcohol is taken in addition to a normal diet, obesity, with all its problems, will result
- Elderly people have an increased tendency to fall, which is aggravated by illness, e.g. stroke or the effects of medication, so superimposing alcohol on top of this will make things worse
- The depressant effect of alcohol on the central nervous system means that nerve impulses take longer to travel to and from the brain. There will be a slowing and dulling of the brain's responses – intoxication. Reactions, thought processes and coordination will suffer. It becomes very difficult to carry out mental and physical tasks, e.g. cooking and cleaning

NB: The blood alcohol level produced by a measured amount of alcohol depends largely upon lean body mass; bone, muscle and organs. The less lean body mass the higher the blood alcohol levels will be. Lean body mass decreases with age.

Women have less lean body mass than men, they also have fewer liver enzymes, therefore, older women are especially sensitive to alcohol.

(Roberts, 1996)

- Alcohol, because of its vasodilation effect, may make an elderly person feel cold
- There will be added dangers if alcohol is mixed with prescribed, or over-the-counter drugs. Elderly people often say they do not drink if taking medicines, but admit to mixing alcohol with over-the-counter drugs (Leach, 1999)

NB: Some medications are likely to cause problems if mixed with alcohol, these include prescriptions for arthritis, anxiety, epilepsy, depression, diabetes, hypotensive agents, antihistamines and antibiotics.

- Alcohol will make worse a failing memory
- Alcohol can increase tension within a relationship or can lead to isolation and/or violence.

An elderly person may not be a heavy drinker, but problems, both physical and psychological, will occur at a low level of drinking.

Symptoms of intoxication

- Mild: Mild euphoria, impairment of judgement, disinhibition, emotional lability
- Moderate: loss of self-control, ataxia, motor discoordination, slurred speech, vomiting, memory loss
- Severe: depression of conscious level, coma, hypertension, acidosis, depression of cough reflex, obstruction of airways.

(Adapted from Taylor, 1998)

Physical problems associated with alcohol abuse

Obesity, malnutrition, pancreatitis, hepatitis, cirrhosis with possible oesophageal varices, hypertension, stroke, cardiomyopathy, osteoporosis, sexual dysfunction, infertility, brain damage, neuropathy, blood clotting deficiencies, frequent accidents, increased likelihood of cancer in the digestive system, liver and breast.

(Adapted from Taylor, 1998)

Answer to question three:
What treatment is available for Mr Ingram?

'Why bother helping him, he's not long for this world, anyway!'
'Alcohol is the only pleasure he has left in life!'
'He doesn't want help, he's happy as he is!'

These are common attitudes towards an elderly drinker and his problems. If alcohol is used sensibly there is no risk of damage to health, so they can be left to drink in peace. Sensible drinking is normal and should be encouraged (Malcolm, 1992).

> **NB:** Alcohol detoxification involves the gradual withdrawal, under cover of medication, of all alcohol. Sudden, complete sobriety will produce unpleasant effects that can be dangerous, especially for elderly people. Relapses are common.
>
> (Roberts, 1988)

Education

- Point out to Mr Ingram the effects of excessive alcohol consumption
- Talk about treatment in a positive way
- Allow time to gain his confidence, perhaps through his son-in-law, Robert
- Respect Mr Ingram's wishes but give advice and information as and when you can. It may be that someone, a professional person, taking an interest in him, will tip the balance towards recovery.

Use of alcohol

Try to persuade Mr Ingram to follow these tips when drinking:

- Take time over drinking. The liver needs, at least, 1 hour to breakdown one unit of alcohol. If he drinks faster than that alcohol will build up in his system, causing intoxification
- Try to keep two or three alcohol-free days each week
- Avoid places where he feels under social pressure to drink
- Stop supplies: whoever does his shopping must reduce the amount of alcohol bought each week
- Mr Ingram should not drink if he is feeling unwell, depressed, overtired or cold
- Eat, as well as drink; never drink on an empty stomach
- Encourage Mr Ingram to have a warm drink at bedtime, rather than an alcoholic one
- Doctors should treat his depression and improve his general health
- Provide company; social support is vital for recovery.

Take time and trouble to get to know Mr Ingram.

He has a choice, but unless he recognises the nature of his problem, he will not be motivated to stop drinking and become socially active, once again.

Answer to question one:
Differentiate between the two approaches used by each nurse.

In the first scenario Caroline, the named nurse, identified that Dorothy was confused. Dorothy's confusion is caused by Alzheimer's disease, but can be exacerbated by pneumonia and a move from her familiar surroundings into hospital. The nurse was trying to make Dorothy understand where she was by orientating her to the present time and place. This is known as reality orientation. The purpose of reality orientation is to 'maintain and improve memory and orientate clients to present day events and activities' (McMahon & Isaacs, 1997, p. 283). It is often used by health care professionals caring for patients with Alzheimer's disease or dementia. Examples may be to begin verbally orientating the patient, writing the day and date next to a clock on a designated chalk board, or informing the patient of what is happening to them and why (Wilcock, 1999).

In this scenario Dorothy was unable to be orientated to reality. Rather she withdrew to the comfort of her past. Due to her confusion about present events and becoming more confused, Dorothy exhibited signs of puzzlement, increasing disorientation and fear. Dorothy was unable to cope with these feelings and became angry and agitated. By trying to get away from the stimuli that caused these feelings, she injured herself by pulling out her cannula.

In the second scenario, Anne the night nurse is aware of Dorothy's confusion. Anne wishes to settle Dorothy and rather than orientate Dorothy, she steps into Dorothy's world. This is known as validation therapy. This was first described by an American social worker named Naomi Feil (1992). Validation means 'to acknowledge the feelings and emotions of the person with dementia, even though the factual content of their conversation is incorrect and meaningless' (McMahon & Isaacs, 1997, p. 29). However although the conversation may be meaningless to the nurse, it has every meaning to the patient. Ultimately this process still enables the health professional to communicate with the person with dementia (Colles & Kydd, 1999). Dorothy may have reverted to speaking to her mum because she feels safe with her in the strange hospital environment. Although the conversation may not seem meaningful to the nurse, the nurse has settled Dorothy and Dorothy's treatment can continue safely. Other patients in the ward will not be further disturbed by Dorothy's actions.

Answer to question two:
Describe and contrast between reality orientation and validation therapy.

The purpose of reality orientation is to try to utilise whatever intellectual ability remains by providing stimulation and exercise to the failing mental capabilities of a person with Alzheimer's disease or a similar condition (Wilcock, 1999). Validation therapy, 'asks the practitioner to respect the world and feelings of the person with dementia and to validate these feelings by focusing upon that person's experiences of the "here and now" ' (Keady, 1999). It must be remembered that the person with dementia's perception of the here and now may be much different to the actual place, day, time and person of the person or people around them. Our reality could differ greatly from the reality that the person with dementia is experiencing.

Validation therapy is person centred and values the patient and their line of thought. Reality orientation is concerned with the here and now and bringing the patient to them.

Answer to question three:
Select several counselling/communication techniques that could be used by the nursing staff to reduce Dorothy's fears.

There are many different techniques and skills that nurses can use to help reduce a patient's fears and anxieties. Several of the commonly used techniques are outlined below.

Empathy

Empathy is a word often heard in nursing. Carl Rogers first termed and defined empathy in 1957. Since then there have been many definitions of the word. A more recent definition of empathy is, 'the ability to understand accurately what another person's world looks and feels like from their point of view and to convey this understanding in a relationship' (Bayne et al, 1998, p. 67).

Empathy should not be confused with sympathy. In empathy the person feels with the person, rather than a sympathetic feeling out of compassion or sorrow for someone.

The benefit of empathy is that it allows the nurse to step into the patient's shoes and see the world as they see it. In Dorothy's case, Anne the night nurse empathised with Dorothy and saw that Dorothy was back in her childhood so she adopted the surrogate role of her mother (Peplau, 1952) to help empathise with Dorothy. Tilbury (1993) refers to this as understanding the other's world, through empathy.

Genuineness

Also referred to as congruence (Bayne et al, 1998, p. 69) and realness (Tschudin, 1991, p. 4). Genuineness requires the nurse to be, 'a real person with the client' and 'not adopt a pose and is as spontaneous and non-defensive as the situation allows,' (Bayne et al, 1998, p. 69).

In the case study, Caroline the nurse remained the nurse, but in Dorothy's eyes was her mum. The nurse did not ask leading questions, but general reflective questions. It would have been easy for the nurse to role play Dorothy's mum, but Caroline would be acting and adopting a pose. Rather Caroline tried to be herself as non-defensively as possible. Although Dorothy became agitated and frightened Caroline tried to pacify her by unsuccessfully orientating her.

In the second scenario, Anne, the night nurse, remained a genuine person, although Dorothy saw her as her mum. Anne's response was to ask questions based on the information given by Dorothy. This was in a non-threatening sincere manner, which put Dorothy at her ease.

Acceptance

Carl Rogers, the psycho-therapy Guru of the 1950s and 1960s referred to this as, 'unconditional positive regard'. Tschudin (1991, p. 5) refers to acceptance as 'warmth'. She further describes warmth as, 'respecting another person, and what that person is and stands for'.

Acceptance, 'implies respect for the other as a person of value and unique worth' (Bayne et al, 1998).

Although the nurses accept Dorothy and what she says, they do not have to believe it as the truth. Thus the nursing staff can value Dorothy as a person and accept what she says, but not believe that they are her mother.

References

Bayne, R., Nicolson, P., Horton, I. (1998). Counselling and communication skills for medical and health practitioners. Leicester: The British Psychological Society.

Colles, S, Kydd, A. (1999). Dementia Services Development Centre: A Practice Guide for Community Nursing. Dementia Touches Everyone, Practice Series No. 2 (2nd ed.). Stirling: The Queen's Nursing Institute, University of Stirling.

Feil, N. (1992). Validation: The Feil method – How to help disorientated old-old. (2nd ed.). Ohio: Edward Feil Productions.

Keady, J. (1999). Dementia. Elderly Care 11(1): 21–27.

McMahon, C., Isaacs, R. (1997). Care of the Older Person. A Handbook for Care Assistants. Oxford: Blackwell Science.

Peplau, H. (1952). Interpersonal Relations in Nursing. New York: G.P. Putman's Sons.

Rogers, C. (1957). A note on 'The Nature of Man.' Journal of Counselling Psychology 4: 199–203.

Tilbury, D. (1993). Working with Mental Illness. London: BASW/Macmillan.

Tschudin, V. (1991). Counselling Skills for Nurses (3rd ed.). London: Baillière Tindall.

Wilcock, G. (1999). Living with Alzheimer's Disease and Similar Conditions. (2nd ed.). London: Penguin Books.

Assessment of elimination status

Penelope Simpson

Floella George, a widow aged 82, has been admitted to respite residential care. She was widowed 20 years ago and has five children, two of whom live nearby. The third lives in Jamaica, Floella's country of origin.

Floella finds it difficult to walk more than 3 m due to her painful knees and hips. She was diagnosed as having rheumatoid arthritis 15 years ago and has been finding it progressively more difficult to mobilise. Her hands are stiff and she has had to give up her favourite hobby of knitting.

She has a good appetite, but has found it difficult to prepare food for herself. Her two closest children usually do her shopping and provide some meals across the week. The others visit regularly. The residential home has been asked to assess her health status in detail.

Question one: How would you assess Floella's elimination status?

15 minutes

Question two: Draw and label two simple diagrams of the main structures involved in elimination.

15 minutes

Time allowance: **30 minutes**

Answer to question one:
How would you assess Floella's elimination status?

Floella's mental status needs to be established as that may be one of the reasons for her admission. If there is significant memory loss, the history taken from her may be unreliable, and supporting information may need to be gained from her daughters (Nazarko, 1997a).

As part of an ongoing assessment process, she needs to be tactfully asked if she has any problems with bladder or bowels, such as pain, constipation, leakage (urine), or soiling (faeces). The assessor will use observation and sense of smell to detect possible incontinence.

Find out her normal pattern of elimination; micturating up to seven times a day and twice a night is normal; defecation up to nine times a day is also normal (Hocking, 1999). Does she suffer from urgency, hesitancy, burning, haematuria? Observe her urine for colour, concentration, clarity and odour. A urinalysis will identify problems such as infection or diabetes (Marjoram, 1999). Healthy urine should be pale and plentiful (Simpson, 1999). What is the consistency of her stools and does she have to strain to defecate?

Are there any barriers to elimination in Floella's usual environment, such as the only toilet being upstairs or outside? Her mobility (for getting to the toilet unaided), and dexterity (to get undressed in time once she gets there), need to be determined to identify any difficulties, and what level of support will be needed (Nazarko, 1997b; Vernon & Bleakley, 1997). Is she already taking any measures to help, such as medication, pelvic floor exercises (Haslam, 1997; Willis, 1997), fluids, diet, pads, electrical stimulation (Bo & Talseth, 1997) or other devices such as cones or weights?

Also check her weight and identify if she has gained or lost any recently. A dietary history could be used to identify the amount of fibre/non-starch polysaccharides (NSPs) in her diet. Lack of NSPs can lead to constipation.

Box 6.1

Non-starch polysaccharides: a collection of indigestible substances found in plant cell walls and not in animal food sources.

   Function: aids the passage of food through the bowel and eases elimination. Recommended daily intake 18 g to reduce constipation, diverticular disease and bowel cancer risk.

   Sources: fruits and vegetables, whole grains, wholemeal bread, cereals, beans and pulses.

Check against the 'tilted plate' for dietary balance (see Joe Church profile; Simpson, 1999). Her body mass index (BMI) should be found by dividing her weight in kilograms by the height in metres squared. Would a reducing/enriched diet be helpful? (Simpson, 1999). Being overweight can alter the angle of the urethra in women and reduce continence.

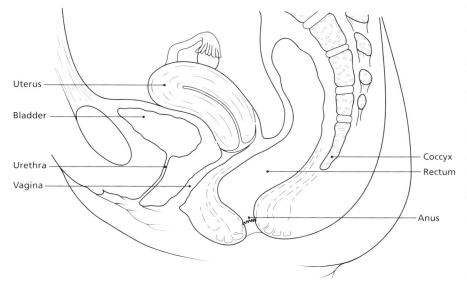

Uterus

Bladder

Urethra

Vagina

Coccyx

Rectum

Anus

Figure 6.1: Side view of pelvis.

What is her fluid intake? It should be 30–35 ml per kilogram body weight per day (Marjoram, 1999). Does it consist of dehydrating fluids such as alcohol, strong tea and coffee, the last of which stimulates the bowel? Excess alcohol can cause diarrhoea. Lack of fluid can lead to cystitis, constipation or kidney stones.

Does she have any health problems or is she taking medication that may have an impact on her elimination? For example diuretics may cause urinary incontinence (Nazarko, 1997a); antacids and analgesic drugs may cause constipation.

Her obstetric history is relevant, as delivering five children may have left her with a weak pelvic floor and stress incontinence (Dowse, 1997). Coughing, laughing, lifting, running or jumping puts pressure on the pelvic floor muscles and causes leakage of urine. Hormone changes during the menopause can cause loss of muscle tone and prolapse of the uterus puts stress on the pelvic floor. A tendency to constipation weakens these muscles and being overweight is a compounding factor. Box 6.2 shows the procedure for pelvic floor exercises.

Box 6.2 Pelvic floor exercises

Procedure and effect
- Sit comfortably with feet on the floor, and legs slightly apart
- Lean forward
- Elbows can be rested on thighs, or arms left hanging down to prevent using buttock muscles
- Draw the muscles of the vagina upwards and inwards
- Hold for 10 seconds
- Relax for 10 seconds
- Repeat this as often as possible across the day
- At first aim at 50/day in blocks of 10
- Set intervals at which to do these, such as immediately after passing urine
- Increase the daily number within the limits of tiredness to 100/day
- It takes 3 months to achieve tangible benefits.

Do
- Aim for contractions of at least 2 seconds
- Visualise stopping a flow of urine to use the right muscles.

Avoid
- Breath holding
- Squeezing buttock muscles
- Tensing the abdomen
- Interrupting urine flow except as a test once a week.

(Willis, 1997)

Answer to question two:
Draw and label two simple diagrams of the main structures involved in elimination.

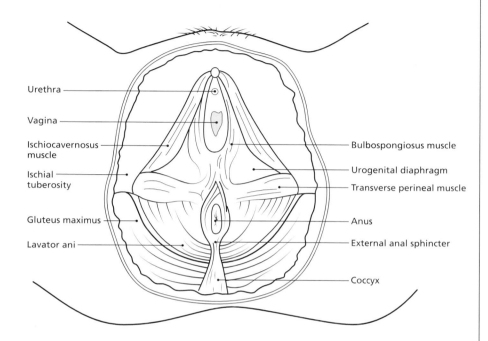

Urethra

Vagina

Ischiocavernosus muscle

Ischial tuberosity

Gluteus maximus

Lavator ani

Bulbospongiosus muscle

Urogenital diaphragm

Transverse perineal muscle

Anus

External anal sphincter

Coccyx

Figure 6.2: Muscles of the pelvic floor.

References

Bo, K., Talseth, T. (1997). Change in urethral pressure during voluntary pelvic floor muscle contraction and vaginal electrical stimulation. Urogynaecology Journal 8: 3–7.

Dowse, J. (1997). Floor plan. Finding the flaw. Nursing Times 93(15): 76.

Haslam, J. (1997). Floor plan. Nursing Times 93(15): 67–70.

Hocking, J. (1999). Continence problems: how to tackle reticence of patients. Nursing Times 95(1): 56–58.

Marjoram, B. (1999). Elimination. In: Hogston, R., Simpson, P. (Eds) Foundations of Nursing Practice. Basingstoke: Macmillan, pp. 133–166.

Nazarko, L. (1997a). The whole story. Nursing Times 93(43): 63–66.

Nazarko, L. (1997b). Educating Elsie. Nursing Times 93(43): 68–71.

Simpson, P. (1999). Eating and drinking. In: Hogston, R., Simpson, P. (Eds) Foundations of Nursing Practice. Basingstoke: Macmillan, pp. 93–132.

Vernon, S., Bleakley, S. (1997). A successful bladder retraining programme. Nursing Times 93(38): 50–51.

Willis, J. (1997). Use it or lose it. Nursing Times 93(15): 70–73.

Further reading

Bo, K., Talseth, T., Holme, I. (1999). Single blind, randomised controlled trial of pelvic floor exercises, electrical stimulation, vaginal cones and no treatment in management of genuine stress incontinence. British Medical Journal 318(7182): 487–493.

Chappiti, U., Jean-Marie, S., Chan, W. (2000). Cultural and religious influences on adult nutrition in the UK. Nursing Standard 14(29): 47–51.

Incontinet, a site for incontinence and pelvic muscle disorders is on: http://www.incontinet.com/[Accessed 2000, April 17].

Khullar, V., Cardozo, L.D., Abbott, D., Anders, K. (1997). GAX collagen in the treatment of urinary incontinence in elderly women: a two year follow up. British Journal of Obstetrics and Gynaecology 104: 96–99.

Johanson, J.F., Lafferty, J. (1996). Epidemiology of faecal incontinence: the silent afflication. American Journal of Gastroenterology 91(1): 33–36.

Miller, J.M., Ashton-Miller, J.A., DeLancey, J.O. (1998). A pelvic muscle pre-contraction can reduce cough-related urine loss in selected women with mild SUI. Journal of the American Geriatric Society 46(7): 870–874.

O'Brien, J. (1996). Evaluating primary care interventions for incontinence. Nursing Standard 10(23): 40–43.

Rigby, D. (1996). Face to face support. Nursing Times 92(41): 84.

Siddle, A. (1997). Cut out the padding. Nursing Times 93(43): 76, 78.

Asthma: triggers and treatment

Chris Pearce

> Torben Sonderby is a 36-year-old man of Danish origin, who has lived in England for a number of years. He met his wife, Gillian, whilst she was on holiday in Skagen, Northern Jutland and he was working in a hotel. He followed her to England and they married a year later. They have two children – Marianne, aged 9 and Mogens, aged 7 – who both have their father's blonde hair and blue eyes.
>
> They live in a three-bedroomed house on a development that was built in the last few years. Torben is disappointed that they were unable to buy a house like the ones he used to live in back in Denmark, with pine flooring already installed. He plans to take up all the carpets in the house and add wooden floors as soon as they can afford it. Both children go to the local primary school, which they love, and they are both bilingual. Gillian takes the children to school on her way to work, as the lunchtime cook at a local pub.
>
> Torben is a civil servant and works for the local government, where he is responsible for the recycling of household waste. The children have a number of pets including a rabbit, a dog and a canary, and although they agreed to care for the animals themselves, when they arrived it soon fell to Dad to clean out the rabbit and canary cages each week. Torben and Gillian both like gardening and badminton, and both belong to the local badminton club, which meets regularly on Thursday nights.
>
> When Torben was a teenager he had hay fever every summer. He also began to notice that he became breathless and wheezy whilst doing exercise at school, and whenever he played handball for his local team. He ignored his symptoms as long as he could, but when he started to wake up every night coughing, he went to see his medical practitioner, who diagnosed asthma and commenced the appropriate treatment. He has always considered his asthma to be mild but recently, after a cold he noticed that he has once again started to wake at night with a cough and chest tightness, and is beginning to worry.

Question one: What is asthma and what triggers might affect Torben's asthma?

15 minutes

Question two: Discuss the treatment Torben may require and why it is necessary to take the medication every day.

10 minutes

Time allowance: **25 minutes**

Answer to question one:
What is asthma and what triggers might affect Torben's asthma?

Asthma is a common condition that involves chronic or long-term inflammation of the airways. Because of this the airways are irritable and can therefore narrow easily in response to a wide range of provoking triggers.

The narrowing of the airways is usually reversible, but in some patients who have had asthma for a long time, the inflammation may lead to a permanent narrowing of the airways. Asthma can occur at any age; for most people the age of onset is before the age of 10 (Crockett, 1993, p. 6).

In the airways of asthmatic patients certain triggers cause bronchospasm, inflammation and mucus production. Asthma can be mild, moderate or severe, intermittent or persistent. The cause of asthma is not completely understood. The symptoms of asthma are a cough, wheezing, chest tightness and shortness of breath.

The triggers that are most commonly found to provoke an asthmatic response are upper respiratory tract infections, house dust mites, animals, pollens and grasses and exercise. A person with asthma will often be sensitive to a number of allergens' (Woolner, 1996, p. 42). In Torben's case an upper respiratory tract infection may have been the trigger, but there are a number of trigger factors that Torben may be affected by as he has animals, he suffers from hay fever and there are more carpets on the floor of his house in England than he was used to in Denmark.

Answer to question two:
Discuss the treatment Torben may require and why it is necessary to take the medication every day.

The treatment Torben may require is regular inhaled therapy, which helps to control asthma. The British Thoracic Society produces guidelines that aid doctors in making appropriate treatment choices (The British Guidelines on Asthma Management, 1997). The inhaled drugs are normally classified as preventers and relievers. Preventers, which are inhaled corticosteroids, work by reducing the amount of swelling and mucus in the airways, preventing the inflammatory response. The mode of action of inhaled corticosteroids is not fully understood but it is known that they can reduce bronchial inflammation and stabilise epithelial damage. The risk of acute attack or of long-term irreversible damage is reduced. 'Inhaled steroids are used solely as prophylactic treatment of asthma. They have no immediate effect on the symptoms of asthma' (McKenzie, 1994, p. 875).

Minor side-effects of inhaled steroid treatment include hoarseness and oral *Candida albicans*. The incidence of this can be reduced by rinsing the mouth after the administration of the inhaled steroid treatment. Examples of preventer inhalers are beclomethasone dipropionate, budesonide and fluticasone propionate.

Relievers open the airways and make it easier to move air in and out of the lungs. These drugs act on the Beta 2 receptors of the sympathetic nervous system and dilate the bronchial smooth muscle, thus opening up the airway. They can either be short or long acting. The short-acting group of relievers are usually taken on an 'as needed' basis as they provide quick relief of symptoms, usually within 5 minutes, and the effect lasts for up to 4 hours.

The goal of treatment for asthma is that it is so well controlled that relievers need only be used on an occasional basis. Patients with very mild asthma may be treated with relievers only.

Long-acting relievers have a slower onset of action and the effects continue for about 12 hours. They are therefore taken on a twice daily basis and are used in conjunction with inhaled steroid treatment, particularly if nocturnal and exercise symptoms are a feature (Fox, 1998, p. 8).

Medication should be taken every day, even when the patient is feeling well. The inhaled corticosteroid keeps the asthma under control and may help to keep the lungs healthy. Regular treatment helps to prevent the asthma symptoms getting worse, both in the long and short term.

References

Crockett, A. (1993). Managing Asthma in Primary Care. London: Blackwell Scientific Publications.

Fox, V. (1998). What is the role of long term B2 agonists? The Asthma Journal 3(1): 7–8.

McKenzie, S. (1994). Drugs used to control asthma. British Journal of Nursing 3(17): 872–880

The British Guidelines on Asthma Management (1997). Thorax 52(1): S1–S21.

Woolner, E. (1996), Understanding asthma. Nursing Standard 11(5): 41–45.

Further reading

Brewin, A.M., Hughes J.A. (1995). Effect of patient education on asthma management. British Journal of Nursing 4(2): 81–101.

Cross, S. (1997). The management of acute asthma. Professional Nurse 12(7): 495–497.

Levy, M., Hilton, S., Barnes, G. (1997). Asthma at Your Fingertips (2nd ed.). London: Class Publishing.

Osman, L. (1996) Guided self-management and patient education. British Journal of Nursing 5(13): 785–789.

Newly diagnosed breast cancer

Carmel Sheppard

> Jill is 56 years old, married, and has two daughters, aged 35 and 37. Although Jill works full time as a secretary, her financial situation has been difficult since her husband, Mike, became unemployed 6 months ago. Since then Mike has been increasingly feeling low and depressed, which Jill has equally found difficult to cope with.
>
> Jill noticed a small lump in her left breast whilst in the shower, and immediately decided to visit her doctor. Jill was aware that her mother had died of breast cancer 1 year after her diagnosis at the age of 57 years, and two aunts had also suffered from breast cancer. Jill had received an invitation to attend the 3-yearly National Breast Screening Programme only 6 months ago, but due to her husband's redundancy, she had not considered this a priority at the time and consequently had not attended.
>
> Jill's GP referred her to the breast clinic at the local hospital. Following further investigations, Jill was told that the mammogram showed a small lump in her breast, and that the cells taken on cytology had confirmed the presence of breast cancer. The surgeon explained the treatment options available to Jill; as the lump was close to the nipple, mastectomy and axillary sampling were advised. Other treatments such as radiotherapy, chemotherapy and endocrine therapy were mentioned, and Jill is now aware that further treatments may be advised depending on her histology results.
>
> Jill was admitted to the surgical ward 2 weeks later and underwent her surgery 5 days ago. She is about to be discharged following a left mastectomy and axillary sampling.

Question one: Discuss the psychological implications of Jill's diagnosis in relation to her cancer and treatment.

30 minutes

Question two: Outline the role of the nurse in offering both psychological care and practical advice whilst Jill is in hospital.

30 minutes

Question three: Highlight the psycho-social issues that both Jill and her family may be concerned about.

30 minutes

Question four: What help and advice might you offer in relation to these psycho-social issues?

30 minutes

Time allowance: **2 hours**

Answer to question one:
Discuss the psychological implications of Jill's diagnosis in relation to her cancer and treatment.

The diagnosis of breast cancer for many patients not only provokes fears about the cancer itself but also fears about treatment and its effects. Approximately 20–40% of women suffer anxiety and depression within the first 2 years post-surgery, and one-third of women report psycho-sexual problems (Maguire, 1994). Breast cancer generally speaking affects one in 12 women. For Jill, breast cancer in particular may have been something she has always feared due to her family history. It is important to remember that only between 2% and 10% of breast cancers are in fact genetically related (Page et al, 1995). However, any woman who has three or more first- or second-degree relatives with breast or ovarian cancer, or with a first-degree relative with breast cancer under the age of 40 might be considered approximately three times more likely to develop breast cancer themselves (White & Mackay, 1997).

Jill may be thinking quite negatively in view of her prior personal experiences of breast cancer with her own mother's death. It is often worth checking with any patient whether they have known anyone who has had breast cancer as often their beliefs about cancer may be closely associated with that experience. Many patients may view a diagnosis of cancer as a death sentence, and some patients will still describe cancer as the 'Big C', with the additional belief that it always leads to a painful, undignified death. The thought that it might be catching may lead the patient to become quite isolated and avoid others; some may also feel guilt about somehow causing it (Fallowfield, 1990). For Jill the latter may be particularly important as she may feel guilt over having not attended her breast screening invitation.

The National Screening programme in this country was set up in 1989 (HMSO, 1986; Blamey et al, 1994). All women between the ages of 50 and 64 are invited for breast screening every 3 years. Experience from other countries has demonstrated a reduction in mortality from breast cancer by up to 30% (HMSO, 1986). The document *Health of the Nation* (HMSO, 1992) targeted a reduction in mortality from breast cancer by 25% by the year 2000 in the UK. The national average acceptance for first-time breast screening is approximately 73.1% (Patnick, 1997); however there are often many reasons given by women for non-attendance of screening, some of which include:

- Lack of knowledge about breast screening, i.e. fear of the mammogram being painful
- Fear of what might be found: of cancer, losing a breast, other treatments, and the impact that cancer might have on their family and social relationships
- Personal health beliefs, i.e. 'it won't happen to me', or a belief that breast cancer cannot be cured anyway, or women who rely entirely on breast self-examination to detect breast cancer
- Fear of radiation from the X-rays
- Difficulties in attendance, i.e. work or other commitments, and lack of time
- Financial difficulties in gaining transport and taking time off work

Answer to question four:
What help and advice might you offer in relation to these psycho-social issues?

- Give the opportunity for Jill to discuss her fears in relation to her daughters. Information such as the availability of family history mammography screening, genetic clinics, genetic testing, and information regarding current research trials such as the tamoxifen prevention trial (which is a national trial currently run in several hospitals) may be helpful. If the daughters have expressed concerns, it may be helpful to include them in this discussion.
- Give Jill the time to talk about her feelings and how she feels her cancer may affect her role within the family. Many patients feel unable to share their underlying fears about the cancer with the family in an attempt to protect the family and not add to their psychological pain.
- Allow Jill to discuss her fears in relation to her husband's depression. She may be excluding her husband from the opportunity to be present at appointments, and also excluding him from the opportunity to talk openly and honestly about their fears together, in an attempt to protect him. For many partners the impact of their spouse's diagnosis may be equal to the impact on the patient (Sheppard & Markby, 1995). It might be helpful to encourage Jill to include Mike, by bringing him to her appointments; obviously for ethical reasons, this must be the patient's choice.
- A further concern for Jill is her financial situation. It may be appropriate to involve the social services to advise if there is any additional help that they are entitled to. It may be also possible to apply for a charity grant, for example, from Macmillan Cancer Relief. A grant might help to cover the costs of any outstanding bills, or mortgage arrears for instance that have arisen as a result of Jill's being unable to work. The breast care nurse or Macmillan nurse may be able to offer further information regarding the availability of grants.

References

Blamey, R., Wilson, A., Patnick, J., Dixon, J. (1994). Screening for breast cancer. British Medical Journal 6961(309): 1076–1079.

Bundred, N., Morgan, D., Dixon, J. (1994). Management of regional nodes in breast cancer. British Medical Journal 6963(309): 1222–1225.

Fallowfield, L. (1990). Quality of Life. London: Routledge.

Fallowfield, L. (1991). Breast Cancer. London: Routledge.

HMSO (1986). Report to the Health Ministers of England, Wales, Scotland and N. Ireland. Working group chaired by Sir Patrick Forrest. Breast Cancer Screening. London: HMSO.

HMSO (1992). A Strategy for Health in England. Health of the Nation. London: HMSO.

Maguire, P. (1994). Psychological aspects. British Medical Journal 6969(309): 1649–1652.

Page, D., Steel, C., Dixon, J. (1995). Carcinoma in situ and patients at high risk of breast cancer. British Medical Journal 6971(310): 39–42.

Patnick, J. (1997). Breast Screening: Review 97. Sheffield: National Health Service Breast Screening Programme.

Rafferty, D. (1995). Body image: using women who have had breast surgery as a case study. International Journal of Palliative Nursing 1(4): 195–199.

Sainsbury, J., Anderson, T., Morgan, D.A.L., Dixon, J. (1994). Breast cancer. British Medical Journal 6962(309): 1150–1153.

Sheppard, C., Markby, R. (1995). The partner's experience of breast cancer: A phenomenological approach. International Journal of Palliative Nursing 1(3): 134–140.

Watson, J., Sainsbury, J., Dixon, J. (1995). Breast reconstruction after surgery. British Medical Journal 6972(310): 117–118.

White, E., Mackay, J. (1997). Genetic screening: risk factors for breast cancer. Nursing Times 93(41): 58–59.

Further reading

Denton, S. (1996). Breast Cancer Nursing. London: Chapman Hall.

Fallowfield, L., Baum, M., Maguire, P. (1986). Effects of breast conservation on psychological morbidity associated with diagnosis and treatment of early breast cancer. British Medical Journal 6558(293): 1331–1334.

Faulder, C. (1995). Breast Cancer and Cancer Care. London: Ward Lock.

Baum, M., Saunders, C., Meredith, S. (1994). Breast Cancer. A Guide for Every Woman. Oxford: Oxford University Press.

Useful addresses

Breast Cancer Care
Kiln House,
210 Kings Road,
London SW6 4NZ
Tel: 0500 245345

BACUP
3 Bath Place,
Rivington Street,
London EC2A 3DR
Tel: 020 7696 9003/020 7613 2121/0808 800 1234

Cancer Relief Macmillan Fund
15/19 Britten Street,
London SW3 3TZ.
Tel: 020 7351 7811.

Cardiac arrest: ventricular fibrillation: relatives in the resuscitation room

Debra Elliot

Rafel Bibi, a 62-year-old widow and mother of five children, is of Indian origin and a Muslim. She lives with her eldest daughter, Meeta, in a small, three-bedroomed town house. Her daughter has three children aged 10–15, who all attend local schools. Rafel's other children all live locally and she sees most of them daily. Rafel is retired and has a small state pension but relies heavily on her family for supplemental income. She enjoys music and sewing but is finding it increasingly difficult to sew as her vision is deteriorating.

Rafel is vegetarian and cooks most of the family meals. She is slightly overweight, has elevated blood pressure for which she takes medication, and is also a tablet-controlled diabetic. Her blood pressure is checked 6-monthly by her GP and she sees the diabetic specialist at 3-monthly intervals.

Rafel has felt 'off colour' the last few days and has been increasingly tired. This morning she has chest pain radiating to her left arm and jaw. Her daughter decides to drive her to the local Casualty department for investigation. Rafel collapses in the backseat on route to the department and on arrival is found to be unresponsive.

Question one: What action should be taken by the nurse on finding Rafel?

15 minutes

Question two: What is ventricular fibrillation and how is it treated?

10 minutes

Question three: Should Rafel's relatives be present during resuscitation?

15 minutes

Time allowance: **40 minutes**

Answer to question one:
What action should be taken by the nurse on finding Rafel?

The nurse needs to safely approach Rafel and establish the result of the collapse. She needs to be quickly moved from the car onto a stretcher or the floor. The nurse is unlikely to be able to manage this herself so should either gain assistance from Rafel's daughter or colleagues in the department. The nurse should then gently shake Rafel's shoulders and shout loudly 'Are you all right?' If there is no response, the nurse should shout for help. Following this the nurse should open Rafel's airway using the head tilt chin lift manoeuvre and ensure the airway is clear by removing any visible obstructions. Then the nurse should check for signs of breathing for up to 10 seconds. This is performed by looking for signs of chest movement, listening for breath sounds and feeling for air on your cheek (Handley et al, 1997).

If Rafel is not breathing, if not already obtained, assistance must be sought. In hospital this is likely to be a cardiac arrest call. Two effective rescue breaths should then be given. To achieve this, the head and chin should be tilted, the nose pinched with the index finger and thumb, and having taken a breath, the nurse's mouth should be placed over Rafel's mouth to ensure a good seal. The nurse should then breathe out slowly over 1.5–2 seconds (in most hospitals,

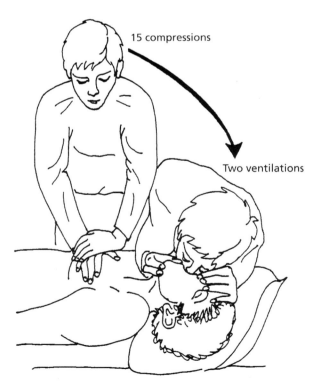

Figure 9.1: Single rescuer resuscitation.

devices are available for airway management and this prevents the need for mouth-to-mouth contact; these include a pocket mask and a bag–valve–mask device).

Having given two rescue breaths, the nurse should check for signs of circulation. This includes checking for any signs of movement and feeling for a carotid pulse; this should take no longer than 10 seconds. If there are no signs of a circulation, chest compressions should be commenced. These are performed by locating the lower half of the sternum and placing the heel of one hand there and the other hand on top of the first. The fingers are interlocked, the arms positioned vertically above the chest and the sternum is compressed 4–5 cm at a rate of 100/minute (Sadik & Elliott, 1999).

Rescue breathing and chest compressions should be combined at a rate of 15 compressions to two breaths for a single rescuer and five compressions to one breath for two rescuers (see Fig. 9.1). In a non-clinical setting, resuscitation should be continued until there are signs of life, help arrives or the rescuers are exhausted (Handley et al, 1997). Within a clinical setting, if resuscitation is not successful, a decision needs to be made whether to continue resuscitation attempts or to abandon them. This is a difficult decision, and is usually made by the most senior clinician present, although increasingly this decision is a team discussion that may involve relatives if they are present. The decision will be made on factors such as the patient's wishes, previous medical condition and quality of life (Royal College of Nursing, British Medical Association and Resuscitation Council (UK), 1993).

Client profiles in nursing: adults & the elderly

Answer to question two:
What is ventricular fibrillation and how is it treated?

Ventricular fibrillation (VF) is random, uncoordinated electrical activity within the ventricles (see Fig. 9.2). Individual muscle fibres are contracting independently and there is no cardiac output, hence a cardiac arrest (Resuscitation Council (UK), 1998). VF is the commonest rhythm during cardiac arrest and requires immediate treatment or cerebral hypoxia will occur rapidly. The definitive treatment of VF is defibrillation. Defibrillation is the delivery of an electrical stimulus (DC shock) to the heart to depolarise myocardial cells in an attempt to restart the heart in sinus rhythm. To be effective, defibrillation must be applied early (Bossaert et al, 1997). Survival is around 90% if patients are defibrillated within 90 seconds of the onset of VF, but this deteriorates to around 1–2% after 20 minutes. Defibrillation is an expanded role in most hospitals for qualified nurses and requires a period of training followed by assessment. When assessed as competent, nurses are usually allowed to deliver three shocks (200 J, 200 J and 360 J) prior to the arrival of a cardiac arrest team. This prompt action obviously markedly increases the patient's chance of survival (Resuscitation Council (UK), 1998).

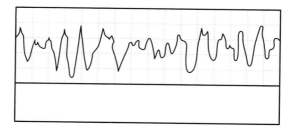

Figure 9.2: Ventricular fibrillation.

Answer to question three:
Should Rafel's relatives be present during resuscitation?

This subject can be highly controversial and there is no right or wrong answer (Walker, 1999). Hospital staff may be unfamiliar with this occurrence and therefore may feel uncomfortable and awkward (although increasingly parents are present during resuscitation attempts on children); whereas paramedics often have relatives or members of the public watching their 'performance' and may feel less intimidated. If Rafel's relatives are present during the resuscitation attempt, someone experienced should be available to stay and support them and to explain what is happening in terminology that is clear and understandable. Ideally they would be away from the stretcher and therefore in no immediate danger themselves, and also not in the way of staff. Throughout the procedure they may change their mind about watching and this should be respected (Resuscitation Council (UK), 1998). If Rafel's relatives are not present throughout the resuscitation attempt, they should be kept constantly informed of the situation. Ideally this is by a member of staff they have already had contact with, although in Casualty departments this is unlikely.

Dealing with distressed relatives is never easy. The following principles recommended by the Resuscitation Council (UK) (1998) may help to ease the situation:

- Prepare yourself and be prepared to spend time with the relatives
- Take someone with you if you are inexperienced
- Confirm that you are speaking to the correct relatives
- Introduce yourself and sit at eye level to the closest relative or friend and look at them when you speak
- Be honest and direct and get to the point quickly
- If their relative has died use the words death or dead not euphemisms
- Be prepared to repeat whatever is necessary and be prepared (and allow) for a range of reactions including anger, denial, numbness, guilt and acute distress.

References

Bossaert, L., Callanan, V., Cummins, R.O. (1997). Early defibrillation. Resuscitation 24: 211–225.

Handley, A.J., Becker, L.B., Allen, M., van Drenth, A., Kramer, E.B., Montgomery, W.H. (1997). Single rescuer adult basic life support. Resuscitation 34: 101–108.

Resuscitation Council (UK) (1998). Advanced Life Support Manual. (3rd ed.) London: Resuscitation Council.

Royal College of Nursing, British Medical Association and Resuscitation Council (UK) (1993). Cardiopulmonary resuscitation – a statement from the Royal College of Nursing, British Medical Association and Resuscitation Council (UK). Royal College of Nursing, British Medical Association and Resuscitation Council (UK).

Sadik, R., Elliott, D.T. (1999). Respiration & circulation. In: Hogstone, R., Simpson, P.M. (Eds) Foundations of Nursing Practice. Basingstoke: Macmillan: pp. 167–215.

Walker, W.M. (1999). Do relatives have a right to witness resuscitation? Journal of Clinical Nursing 8(6): 625–630.

Client profiles in nursing: adults & the elderly

Further reading

Brummel, S. (1998). Resuscitation in the A&E department: can concepts of death aid decision making? Accident & Emergency Nursing 6(2): 75–81.

Phillips, K. (1999). The decision to resuscitate: older people's views. Journal of Clinical Nursing 8(6): 753–761.

Resuscitation Council (UK) (1997). The 1997 Resuscitation guidelines for use in the United Kingdom. London: Resuscitation Council.

Stein–Parbury, J. (1993). Patient and Person – Developing Interpersonal Skills in Nursing. London: Churchill Livingstone.

Wright, B. (1996). Sudden Death – Intervention Skills. (2nd ed.) London: Churchill Livingstone.

Communual living: hearing loss: care of a hearing aid

Vivienne Mathews

Mrs Rodenhever is a resident of the Arcacia House Rest Home, where she has been living for the past 2 months. Mrs Rodenhever is 90 years old and has, up until now, lived on her own since the death of her husband 28 years ago.

She is bright and intelligent, with a fund of funny stories to tell about her life and girlhood growing up in the New Forest.

Increasingly, she is having problems coming to terms with her deafness. She feels isolated, dependent and cut off from her former life. She likes to sit in the day room of the rest home, but although she can see everyone coming and going, she feels lonely as her hearing aid is, inevitably, turned off; the television is always on and no one takes any notice of her.

At coffee time, Mrs Rodenhever is asked if she would like a drink. She says she can't hear what is being said, so the nurse turns on Mrs Rodenhever's hearing aid and speaks very loudly directly into it. Mrs Rodenhever gets agitated and tries to push the nurse away, saying 'How dare you shout at me!'

Question one: Describe the ageing changes that may alter an elderly person's ability to discriminate between sounds.

10 minutes

Question two: What problems with communal living can you identify for Mrs Rodenhever?

10 minutes

Question three: How may Mrs Rodenhever be helped to feel less isolated and cut off from other people?

10 minutes

Time allowance: **30 minutes**

Answer to question one:
Describe the ageing changes that may alter an elderly person's ability to discriminate between sounds.

Deafness is a common, but not inevitable, accompaniment of ageing. There is a general deterioration in the auditory system with age, leading to the following functional changes:

- Loss of the ability to locate sounds
- Narrowing of the range of audible frequencies, with an increased loss in the higher registers

> **NB:** By the age of 60, three-quarters of the capacity to hear high frequency sounds are lost. One-third of people over the age of 65 suffer hearing loss to the point that it interferes with their lives.
> (Christiansen & Grzybowski, 1993)

- Ear wax can cause hearing loss

> **NB:** It is only when ear wax totally occludes the ear canal that perceptible hearing loss occurs. The more impacted the wax (cerumen) the higher the content of keratin and the more the sound is impeded, but partial blockage of the canal by wax can interfere with the satisfactory use of hearing aids.

- Perception of sound may be difficult, especially against a noisy background. This is known as discrimination
- Loudness recruitment: this means that sounds become disproportionately louder to the deaf person, as they increase in intensity (Bond et al, 1993)

> **NB:** Presbycusis is the term used to describe hearing loss in ageing. It is the result of wear and tear of the cells in the inner ear that respond to sound waves. Excessive noise in earlier life, over a prolonged period, may predispose to this type of hearing loss in later life.

- Presbycusis also causes sound localisation problems, making it difficult to tell the direction from which a sound is coming.

Changes associated with deafness

- Impaired reflex posture control
- Uncertainty and unreliability in moving about in the darkness, because of degeneration in the semi-circular canals
- Rapid speech or complex instructions are not understood.

Answer to question two:
What problems with communal living can you identify for Mrs Rodenhever?

The term 'communal environment' can be used to identify many situations, such as long-stay wards, nursing homes, boarding schools, cruise liners, and prisons. The list is long, but the main fact is that a person is living with other people for 24 hours each day.

Goffman (1966) writes that living in an institution puts the three areas of human interaction – work, rest and play – under one governing body; one central control, to the detriment of inmates and their guardians.

Moving into a communal environment involves many changes, so a person's decision to give up his or her own home is not to be taken lightly.

There are, of course, positive reasons for living with others: the end of loneliness or isolation, no more worries about shopping, cooking, cleaning, laundry etc. These factors may far outweigh the negative aspects of institutional care, e.g. eating food not of your choosing, at the wrong time of day for you, or having relative strangers deal with intimate parts of your body.

> **NB:** Isolation is a major problem for many elderly deaf people.
> (Greene & Mosher-Ashley, 1997)

In Mrs Rodenhever's case, living with others is a mixed blessing, as it has given her freedom from daily chores, yet has brought into prominence her hearing problems, which have a severe impact on her ability to adjust to her new home and communicate with those around her. The television is always on, creating background noise, over which she cannot distinguish individual sounds.

> **NB:** Hearing loss does not decline equally across the sound spectrum. It is greater for high-pitched sounds than for low-pitched sounds. Vowels tend to be heard, but not consonants, so that 'I can hear you speaking, but can't tell what you are saying!' is the case.
> (Brooks, 1993)

Mrs Rodenhever turns her hearing aid off as she enters the television lounge, as it not only amplifies speech directed at her, but amplifies all other sounds as well, making it impossible for her to discriminate between general noise and specific sounds.

Answer to question three:
How may Mrs Rodenhever be helped to feel less isolated and cut off from other people?

Mrs Rodenhever feels that her independence has been compromised. She has to be allowed to grieve for the loss of her home, belongings, former lifestyle and for her hearing loss. As yet, she has not settled into her new environment, where everything is strange and no one appears to have any time for her. The routines are new, the people she sees every day are strangers and the layout of the home is still alien to her.

Time will change a lot of these impressions as routines, personnel and the environment become more familiar to her.

It would be helpful if the television was turned off, as low-frequency background noise will conceal higher frequency sounds, such as speech. Residents then may have the opportunity to communicate with each other and let programmes selected by the residents be the order of the day, or to find a quiet spot so that Mrs Rodenhever can have her hearing aid on and interact with others without extraneous background noise (Meecham, 1999).

Speech should be clear and slightly slowed so that clarity of speech is increased. Do not speak too slowly, as this will give the impression that the recipient is stupid or mentally impaired.

Visual clues, such as lip reading, are important. Do not overemphasise lip and tongue movements as this will distort the natural shape of the mouth when using consonants.

It would help Mrs Rodenhever if she were face-to-face, at a comfortable 1 m away and on the same level with whoever is communicating with her (Meecham, 1999).

When communicating with Mrs Rodenhever, her full name should be used first of all, as this will attract her attention.

It would be a very good idea to check Mrs Rodenhever's hearing aid. For a diagram of the parts of a hearing aid, see Agnes Rivendale's profile (p. 137)

Care of a hearing aid

- Wipe the mould, microphone and tubing with a soft tissue
- Do not dampen/wet the microphone
- Wash tubing and mould in warm, soapy water, rinse and dry thoroughly
- Expel water from the tubing by blowing down it
- Tubing should be changed every 6 months
- Batteries last about 1 month. A new supply of batteries should be on hand
- Remove batteries from the hearing aid when not in use for a long period, as they leak
- Batteries are small and can be easily lost; put them somewhere safe
- Training and encouragement may be needed to get the most out of a hearing aid.

An introductory leaflet, as a welcome to the home could be a useful way of imparting vital information, e.g. who's who on the staff, meal times, religious service times etc. A resident such as Mrs Rodenhever will not want to be bombarded with details all at once, but various points should be discussed over the first few days. The sooner she discovers what she needs to know about her new home, the sooner she can relax and start to feel comfortable.

Use equipment, such as assistive listening devices, signalling, alarms and telecommunications to help communicate with Mrs Rodenhever. When speaking with her, adopt a comfortable position, on the same level as her and in which eye contact can be made. Talk slowly, clearly and without the use of jargon. Watch for non-verbal clues that she has understood and ask questions to ascertain the amount of understanding she has of any situation (Shepherd, 1994).

Training should be extended to all staff and should be designed to foster awareness and understanding of the social and psychological stresses that may be associated with hearing loss.

Establish trust and rapport with Mrs Rodenhever, in order to enhance her quality of life in the rest home environment.

References

Bond, J., Coleman, P., Peace, S. (1993). Ageing in Society: An Introduction to Social Gerontology. (2nd ed.). London: Sage Publications Ltd.

Brooks, D. (1993). Hearing aids. In: Bond, J., Coleman, P., Peace, S. Ageing in Society: An Introduction to Social Gerontology. (2nd ed.). London: Sage Publications Ltd.

Christiansen, J., Grzybowski, J. (1993). Biology of Aging. St Louis, MO: Mosby Yearbook, Inc.

Goffman, I. (1996). Asylums. Middlesex: Penguin.

Greene, A.W., Mosher-Ashley, P.M. (1997). A residential care alternative for elderly deaf people. Journal of Gerontological Nursing August 1997.

Meecham, E. (1999). Audiology and hearing impairment: improving the quality of care. Nursing Standard 13(43): 42–46.

Shepherd, M. (1994). Royal National Institute for Deaf People. Training Development Division Leaflet. London: Royal National Institute for the Deaf.

Useful addresses

Hearing Concern. (Formerly the British Association of the Hard of Hearing. BAHOH.)
7/11 Armstrong Road
London W3 7JL
Tel: 020 8743 1110

Hearing Aid Council
Moorgate House
201, Silbury Boulevard
Central Milton Keynes
Bucks MK4 1LZ
Tel: 01908 585442

Community discharge: health promotion

Penelope Simpson (from an outline by Iris Joly)

Doris Gaudion, aged 64, lives on her own in a second floor council flat, which she shared with her husband until his sudden death from a heart attack 9 months ago. The flats are on the edge of a large estate about 3 miles from the town centre. There is one town bus an hour and the service finishes in the early evening. Doris would like to be able to change her accommodation as she is finding the stairs increasingly difficult to climb; she would also like to have a cat to keep her company. Her present accommodation does not allow her to have a pet. Since her husband's death, Doris has become quite isolated; she does not have many friends and has few other interests apart from knitting and watching the television.

Doris has one daughter, Jane, who lives 20 miles away and visits whenever she can. Jane, who is a single parent, works full time as a shop assistant and has two teenage boys. Doris feels her daughter has quite a difficult time so she does not want to bother her, but is happy to see Jane whenever she can visit.

Doris was admitted to hospital for observations after falling and hitting her head on an icy pavement. She sustained bruising to the left side and her forehead; there were no bone injuries. Apart from a persistent slightly raised blood pressure, all other neurological observations were satisfactory. A physical examination detected no other obvious problems.

On admission there was a slight trace of glucose in her urine, which was not there at subsequent testing. Her body mass index of 27.5 supported the observation that Doris was obese. While on the ward she had been very quiet and appeared reluctant to move, becoming a little breathless on exertion. She did not appear to be interested in talking to the other patients and was initially quite happy for the nurses to do most things for her. She needed encouragment to be self-caring.

Question one: When planning Doris' discharge, which health promotion issues should be considered and why?

10 minutes

Question two: What advice should be given to Doris?

10 minutes

Question three: Which members of the multidisciplinary team could be involved? Briefly describe their roles in maintaining her progress.

10 minutes

Time allowance: **30 minutes**

Answer to question one:
When planning Doris' discharge, which health promotion issues should be considered and why?

The most obvious problem for Doris is her obesity. This could be implicated in her slightly elevated blood pressure and the evidence of glucose in her urine. Her obesity increases her chances of a cerebrovascular accident (CVA) (DOH, 1991; 1998), and as such is a government target for health promotion initiatives such as *Health of the Nation* (1991) and *Our Healthier Nation* (1998). There is also a risk of late onset diabetes (Avery, 1998).

Another health promotion topic is exercise. Doris' lifestyle could indicate a lack of exercise, which could exacerbate the obesity (Wakefield, 1999; O'Brien, 2000). Her breathlessness could be due to obesity as no other obvious physical cause was found.

The possibility that Doris is depressed after her husband's death should not be overlooked. Her wish to have a pet could indicate feelings of loneliness. If she is depressed, this factor could have a direct effect on the obesity and lack of exercise. The obesity could also contribute to her depression (Thomas, 1998).

Before any intervention is carried out, an assessment of her diet, general lifestyle and mental state should be undertaken and then appropriate advice can be given in an acceptable manner. The history of her obesity is important. Has Doris' weight increase been recent or has this been an ongoing problem? Her knowledge of what constitutes a balanced diet should be ascertained. Her salt intake could need to be assessed in light of her hypertension, especially if she consumes mostly processed foods. Other factors that could influence her diet are education, income, availability of shops, problems with shopping and transport. The way in which she has coped with her bereavement could also be relevant. Personal preferences are an important consideration as is possible alcohol consumption. Alcohol consumption in the elderly and in women is on the increase (Simpson, 1996). This could be contributing to Doris' excess calorie intake and her depression, as alcohol is classified as a depressant drug.

Answer to question two:
What advice should be given to Doris?

Initially advice centred on diet will probably be the most suitable. Bearing in mind the assessment, it could be suggested a diet diary is kept to see where changes could be made.

Using a strategy such as 'the tilted plate' (Simpson, 1999) could be a useful way of explaining a balanced diet (see Joe Church (p. 253) and Fiona McFee (p. 223) profiles). It may be appropriate to give information on essential food groups and their primary function:

- Protein – growth and cell renewal
- Carbohydrates – energy
- Fats – energy
- Vitamins – growth and metabolism
- Minerals – growth and metabolism
- Water – kidney function and waste elimination
- Fibre – prevention of constipation.

Depending on Doris' needs, a range of topics could be discussed to include the different types of fats and their food sources, different types of carbohydrates, monitoring salt and alcohol intake and preparation of budget meals. A range of leaflets could be used to reinforce advice given.

The intention is to get her eat a healthy diet, rather than 'going on a diet', which has been shown to be less effective (Adami et al, 1996) and could well redistribute her weight from a relatively healthy pear shape, to a more risky apple shape (Lean et al, 1998). The most weight Doris should lose is 1 kg/week (2.2 lb). She needs to remember that muscle is heavier than fat, so if her increased activity levels lower her body fat percentage, increasing her muscle mass, she will lose weight more slowly.

Increasing Doris' general activity levels and suitable exercise should be discussed. Her GP may be able to prescribe a fitness assessment and programme if these are available and accessible. The cost of travel to her local leisure centre and suitable fitness sessions need to be considered. If Doris is feeling isolated and would like more social contact, this could be a way of helping her to meet other people. Local provision of suitable sessions needs to be ascertained, otherwise her expectations could be raised and not met.

The level of exercise to be achieved is a minimum of 30 minutes, 5 days/week. During this time, Doris should get warm, sweaty and slightly breathless, but be able to hold a conversation (O'Neill, 1999). Initially, she should be encouraged just to go for short walks; no special equipment is needed, except for comfortable shoes. She could, for instance, walk to the next bus stop, not the nearest. These walks should increase in length and intensity as she gets fitter. She should aim to be able to walk the 3 miles into the town centre in less than 1 hour. Exercise has been shown to improve mood and self-esteem (Chamberlain, 1999; O'Neill 1999), and can suppress the appetite slightly in some people. These effects could enhance her motivation to persist with her lifestyle changes. Perhaps the family could go for a walk together when Jane visits with her sons.

Answer to question three:
Which members of the multidisciplinary team could be involved? Briefly describe their roles in maintaining her progress.

A range of professionals in the community could be relevant to Doris' needs. Their roles are as follows:

1. The *practice nurse* to monitor and advise accordingly on:
   - Blood pressure
   - Urine for glucose
   - Weight loss
   - Dietary changes
   - Exercise achieved.

2. The *GP*, in collaboration with the practice nurse to prescribe suitable treatment, possibly in the form of medication for control of raised blood pressure or hyperglycaemia, but also in the form of exercise sessions, relaxation sessions or counselling for bereavement, if appropriate.

3. *NHS psychologists/counsellors/RMNs* for specialist bereavement counselling.

4. The *social worker* to assist in an application for rehousing. This could also involve the medical team if it is felt there are medical grounds for rehousing; mental health reasons would also be relevant.

5. *Support groups* such as CRUSE or other bereavement counsellors; Help the Aged (see Useful addresses) may be useful in providing support and contact for Doris.

6. *Housing officer.*

7. *Community dietitian.*

References

Adami, G.F., Gandolfo, P., Scopinaro, N. (1996). Binge eating in obesity. International Journal of Obesity 20: 793–794.

Avery, I. (1998). A weight off her shoulders. Nursing Times 94(35): 76–79.

Chamberlain, C. (1999). Mental gymnastics. ABCNEWS [Online]. Available: http://abcnews.go.com/sections/living/InYourHead/allinyourhead.html [Accessed 1999, June 25].

DOH (1991). The Health of the Nation – A Strategy for Health in England. Cmnd 1986. London: HMSO.

DOH (1998). Our Healthier Nation. London: The Stationary Office.

Lean, M.E.J., Han, T.S., Seidell, J.C. (1998). Impairment of health and quality of life in people with large waist circumference. The Lancet 351(9106): 853–856.

O'Brien, C. (2000). Dieting fads: the facts. Nursing Times 96(1): 46–47.

O'Neill, P. (1999). Walking back to healthiness. Nursing Standard 14(4): 14–15.

Simpson, P. (1996). Therapeutic use of alcohol in the elderly. In: Bonner, A., Waterhouse, J. (Eds) Addictive behaviour: molecules to mankind. Basingstoke: Macmillan: pp. 278–279.

Simpson, P.M. (1999). Eating and drinking. In: Hogston, R., Simpson, P.M. (Eds) Foundations of Nursing Practice. Basingstoke: Macmillan: pp. 93–132.

Thomas, D. (1998). Managing obesity: the nutritional aspects. Nursing Standard 12(18): 49–55.
Wakefield, S. (1999). The big issue. Nursing Standard 13(51): 16–17.

Further reading

Ewles L., Simnett, I. (1995). Promoting Health: A Practical Guide. (3rd ed.). London: Scutari Press.
Gray, J., Buttriss, J. (1993). Obesity and weight management (Fact file No. 4). London: National Dairy Council.
Naidoo, J., Wills, J. (1994). Health Promotion Foundations for Practice. London: Baillière Tindall.
Naval Aerospace Medical Institute (1991). Obesity. United States Naval Flight Surgeon's Manual: (3rd ed.) Ch. 5: Internal Medicine: Section IV: metabolic disorders. [Online]. Available: http://www.vnh/FSM/05/04eObesity.html [Accessed 2000, March 2].
O'Meara, S., Glenny, A.M. (1997). What are the best ways of tackling obesity? Nursing Times 96(35): 50–51.

Useful address

Help The Aged: Head Office
St James's Walk
Clerkenwell Green
London EC1R 0BE
Email: infor@helptheaged.org.uk
Website http://www.helptheaged.org.uk

Congestive cardiac failure

Bernard Mark Garrett

Patrick Walker is a 68-year-old man who lives alone, except for the company of his cat, in a semi-detached house in a large northern city. His wife died from breast cancer 2 years ago after several years of treatment for the disease.

Patrick is now retired but used to work as chief mechanic for the city bus company, and has several friends who still work at the depot. He manages to look after himself, cook his own meals and do his own housework.

He has a 35-year-old daughter, Sarah, who lives locally with her husband and their two children. Sarah looks after her young children on a full-time basis but frequently drops in to see her father and takes a keen interest in his welfare. Occasionally she cooks dinner for him or helps him out with household chores. Patrick enjoys a close relationship with his two grandchildren and often takes them out for visits to the park and other local amenities.

Patrick's main hobby is restoring vintage motorcycles, of which he has three. At present he still rides them but is doing so less frequently as he finds manhandling them more difficult of late. He also has a small car, which he uses for trips to the shops, although his daughter is worried about his eyesight and tries to dissuade him from using it.

He has been a smoker for most of his life and currently smokes about 20 cigarettes a day, despite warnings from his doctor and a previous myocardial infarction (MI) of his anterior left ventricle 18 months ago (see Fig. 12.1).

He drinks alcohol in moderation and enjoys a regular pint at the bus depot social club with his friends every Friday night.

His health has not been good since the demise of his wife and he has been taking diuretics to control mild oedema since his MI.

At 4.30 p.m. on a Tuesday afternoon, Patrick's daughter called out his GP as Patrick became acutely breathless and was suffering with abdominal discomfort and gross oedema of his legs.

His GP admitted him to the City Hospital, where a provisional diagnosis of congestive cardiac failure was made by the medical team.

Upon admission, his symptoms include: dyspnoea and cyanosis, oedema of the sacrum and legs, abdominal pain, and a tachycardia of 120 b.p.m. His blood pressure is 120/40 mmHg and he is apyrexial. His daughter has accompanied him to the hospital and he is extremely anxious about his admission.

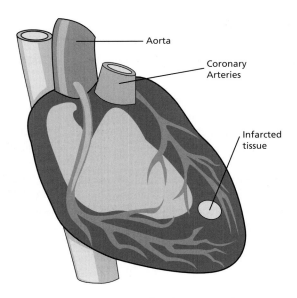

Figure 12.1: Cardiac hypertrophy.

Question one: What underlying pathophysiological changes are likely to have caused Patrick's present problems?

10–15 minutes

Question two: What care should the nurse plan for Patrick for the next 48 hours of his hospitalisation?

15–20 minutes

Time allowance: **25–35 minutes**

Answer to question one:
What underlying pathophysiological changes are likely to have caused Patrick's present problems?

Pulmonary oedema

This is a result of chronic left ventricular failure. As Patrick's left ventricle was damaged by a previous MI, it would be less efficient as a pumping mechanism, resulting in back pressure and congestion of the pulmonary circulation. The increased intravascular pressure in the pulmonary circulation would lead to fluid accumulation in the alveoli (pulmonary oedema, see Fig. 12.2). This would cause his breathlessness (dyspnoea), which would be aggravated by the further cardiac compensatory mechanisms outlined later.

Systemic venous congestion

Systemic oedema would result from combined left and right ventricular heart failure. Patrick's right ventricle will have had to work harder to overcome this congestion and will have compensated by enlarging (hypertrophy, see Fig. 12.2).

Eventually, this compensatory hypertrophy would not have been sufficient to overcome the cardiac workload and right-sided heart failure would have occurred. The resulting increased venous congestion of the systemic circulation would have led to oedema, most noticeable in dependent areas such as Patrick's ankles and sacrum. This is the true technical definition of congestive cardiac failure (Walsh, 1997, p. 364).

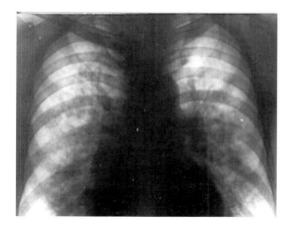

Figure 12.2: Cardiac hypertrophy and pulmonary oedema.

Client profiles in nursing: adult & the elderly

Patrick's body will have initially compensated for the decreased cardiac output following his MI in several ways (Letterer et al, 1992).

Initially his lowered cardiac output and blood pressure would have resulted in increased sympathetic nervous stimulation triggered by baroreceptors in the aortic arch and carotid arteries. This would have increased his heart rate and cardiac contractility, and triggered peripheral vasoconstriction.

Decreased perfusion of the kidneys would also have resulted in activation of the renin–angiotensin mechanism.

This would have caused further vasoconstriction and sodium reabsorption in the kidneys under the influence of aldosterone (released by the adrenal cortex under stimulation by angiotensin II) (Carola et al, 1992, p. 532).

Peripheral vasoconstriction would have increased cardiac afterload (blood volume and arterial resistance) and reduced stroke volume (volume of blood ejected per systolic contraction), resulting in the maintenance of Patrick's blood pressure. However a retention of sodium and fluid in the body will also have resulted primarily from the action of aldosterone (Wilson & Waugh, 1996, p. 222).

The resulting increase in intravascular volume would have caused an increased end-diastolic volume and therefore cardiac preload. This would have helped Patrick maintain normal cardiac filling and cardiac output; it is known as the Frank–Starling mechanism (Letterer et al, 1992), which works up to an extent after which the myocardial fibres become overstretched and cardiac output drops. This would have been attenuated to some extent in Patrick by an increased release of atrial natriuretic peptide (ANP), which is secreted by the atrial walls in response to atrial distention (with congestion). ANP acts on the kidney, increasing sodium excretion and diuresis.

Ventricular hypertrophy would also have occurred in Patrick as a progressive response to increasing fluid volume overload. This type of volume overload results in cardiac wall thickening and an increase in chamber size (eccentric hypertrophy).

The result of this action would be enlargement of the myocardial cells and to an extent improved cardiac contractility.

However, all of these compensatory mechanisms have eventually become exhausted, known as cardiac decompensation, leading to his current condition.

Portal venous congestion

This would also be a result of congestive cardiac failure. It would have caused portal venous hypertension, liver engorgement, abdominal discomfort and possibly ascites (fluid collecting in the peritoneal cavity).

Answer to question two:
What care should the nurse plan for Patrick for the next 48 hours of his hospitalisation?

Physical

The relief of dyspnoea due to pulmonary congestion/oedema and decreased cardiac output is a priority. Sitting him in an upright position to maximise postural drainage and inflation of the lungs will help achieve adequate ventilation (the orthopnoeic position).

He should sleep propped up with pillows to help alleviate nocturnal dyspnoea. Oxygen should be administered as prescribed (normally 40–50%) to improve gaseous exchange and tissue oxygenation. This will reduce the cardiac workload. Oxygen should be humidified to prevent a dry mouth. Smoking should not be permitted as it will exacerbate his dyspnoea and is hazardous in the presence of oxygen. Respiratory rate and depth should be monitored hourly initially.

Due to his impaired cardiac status, cardiac workload should be minimised to prevent exhaustion. Patrick should remain resting in bed with his oxygen therapy (Ryan, 1990). He should be assisted with his hygiene and with commode use when necessary rather than walking any distance.

His cardiac status needs to be monitored carefully with hourly blood pressure and pulse taken initially. If he shows signs of any cardiac dysrythmias, then continuous cardiac monitoring should be instigated.

A full 12-lead electrocardiograph (ECG) should be performed or arranged in order to assess cardiac status and exclude a further MI.

The doctor should prescribe digoxin if Patrick shows signs of atrial fibrillation, which slows the conduction of electrical impulses though the atrioventricular node, slowing the heart rate and improving contractility.

The nurse should administer digoxin as prescribed but only if the pulse rate exceeds 60 b.p.m. as toxicity and bradycardia can develop. Other cardiac inotropes (drugs that improve myocardial contractility) such as dobutamine or dopamine and vasodilators such as isorbide mononitrate may help improve cardiac output (Ryan, 1990). These should be administered as prescribed, and Patrick observed for side-effects, such as hypotension or tachycardia.

Visitors should be advised not to come in large groups or spend too long so as to avoid tiring Patrick.

Oedema due to systemic and pulmonary venous congestion will require careful management. Intravenous (IV) diuretics are likely to be required initially (usually frusemide) to relieve fluid overload (Letterer et al, 1992). The nurse should assist or perform IV cannulation (depending upon skill level and the local policy) and prescribed IV diuretics should be administered by the nurse (or physician depending upon the local IV drug administration policy).

A fluid restriction will be prescribed, usually 1 L in 24 hours at first (Nettina, 1996, p. 310). The nurse should instigate 24-hour fluid balance monitoring, recording all fluid intake and diuresis hourly. A couple of urine bottles should be provided for Patrick immediately and he should be weighed upon admission.

A daily weight chart should also be commenced to monitor daily fluid balance status. Patrick's legs should be kept horizontal on the bed to help alleviate ankle oedema by promoting venous return. However, they should not be raised as this will increase cardiac workload. Patrick should have his oral diuretic dose reviewed by the physicians and this should be administered as prescribed. A low-sodium diet is likely to be necessary to help prevent fluid retention and the dietician should be involved to advise Patrick (Nettina, 1996, p. 310).

Patrick's abdominal discomfort should be alleviated with the resolution of his oedema and venous congestion.

Small meals should be ordered and Patrick encouraged to eat small amounts regularly rather than large meals. If a large volume of ascitic fluid is present, the doctor may perform abdominal paracentesis to drain it. The nurse should assist the doctor in this case and ensure that Patrick understands the procedure. Non-opiate analgesics may be prescribed and given but the nurse should be aware that these are likely to increase the risk of constipation with bed rest.

Patrick has a high risk of pressure ulcer formation due to his impaired peripheral tissue oxygenation and oedema. He should be assessed using a pressure area assessment tool upon admission, such as the Norton Scale (Norton et al, 1975), and have his position changed 2 hourly. A pressure-reducing mattress would also be a useful precaution on his bed.

Patrick is at considerable risk of deep vein thrombosis (DVT) due to decreased cardiac output and bed rest. He should be encouraged to perform limb exercises hourly and have passive limb exercises given 2 hourly if he is unable to do so. A referral to the physiotherapist is also appropriate for daily exercises. Venous compression stockings and a low-dose daily subcutaneous heparin injection would be advisable. This may be prescribed prophylactically whilst Patrick is on bed rest. The nurse should administer this as prescribed (Clagett et al, 1995).

Patrick should have his temperature monitored 4 hourly, as, with pulmonary oedema, the risk of respiratory infection is increased.

Psychological and/or spiritual

Patrick's anxiety will increase the release of adrenaline and sympathetic nervous activity, resulting in increased cardiac workload and thus exacerbating his symptoms.

The nurse should minimise his anxiety by ensuring that all procedures are explained to him, and he understands the reason for his admission. Both Patrick and his relatives should be given the opportunity to voice any concerns or questions they may have to the nurse.

Patrick will be familiar with hospitals due to his wife's previous admission and may have negative feelings about his prognosis. His illness should be carefully explained to him so that he has no illusions about the seriousness of his condition, but is aware that with medication and adapting his lifestyle somewhat, he can improve the quality of his life for a number of years to come.

The opportunity to meet with a religious minister should be arranged if desired by Patrick.

His daughter should be involved to ensure that arrangements are made to look after his house and cat whilst he is hospitalised. His daughter may volunteer to do this, but Social Services or the Royal Society for the Protection of Cruelty to Animals (RSPCA) can be involved if this is not possible.

References

Carola, R., Harley, J.P., Noback, C.R. (1992). Human Anatomy and Physiology. (3rd ed.). New York: McGraw-Hill Inc.

Clagett, G.P., Anderson, F.A., Levine, M.N. (1995). Prevention of venous thromboembolism. Chest 108(4): 312S–334S.

Letterer, R., Carew, B., Reid, M., Woods, P. (1992). Learning to live with congestive heart failure. Nursing 22(5): 34–41.

Nettina, S.M. (Ed.) (1996). Lippincott Manual of Nursing Practice. New York: Lippincott.

Norton, D., McLaren, R., Exton-Smith, A. (1975). An investigation of geriatric nursing problems in hospital. London: Churchill Livingstone. (Original work published in 1962). An investigation of geriatric nursing problems in hospitals. London: National Corporation for the care of old people: 1962.

Ryan, D. (1990). Congestive heart failure: the school of 1990. Care of the Critically Ill 6(2): 38–39.

Walsh, M. (Ed.) (1997). Watson's Clinical Nursing & Related Sciences 5th Ed. London: Baillière Tindall.

Wilson, K.J.W., Waugh, A. (1996). Anatomy and Physiology in Health and Illness. London: Churchill Livingstone.

Further reading

Taylor, C., Lillis, C., LeMone, P. (Eds) (1997). Fundamentals of Nursing: the Art and Science of Nursing Care. Cheltenham: Stanley Thornes Ltd. (Lippincott).

Answer to question two:
Discuss choice in relation to the patient with dementia.

All elderly patients are entitled to live their lives with the same civil and human rights as the rest of the population (Department of Health, 1989). One human right that is particularly important for elderly patients is choice. Iliffe et al (1998, p. 31) define choice as the 'opportunity to select independently from a range of options.'

Although an elderly patient's choice should be respected, one must question how far such a choice should be extended to patients with dementia. Patients with dementia will have a reduced perception and a reduced scope for consent (Hopker, 1999). Keady & Williams (1998) also describe behavioural and personal awareness loss. These factors will consequently affect elderly patients' ability to make informed decisions and choice.

In Mr James's case, his advanced dementia will cause an inability to comprehend his current situation and to act upon information in order to reach an informed decision. However, as with all patients, Mr James should still be informed about decisions regarding his care and preference sought. Decisions and choice may have to be sought from the patient's family.

Client profiles in nursing: adults & the elderly

Answer to question three:
Explain the importance of the role of advocacy in Mr James's situation.

'The word advocacy stems from the Latin verb "advocare", which means to summon, to call for help or to advise. In Roman times this verb had strong legal connections and connotations' (McMahon & Isaacs, 1997, p. 81).

In nursing, advocacy has been described by Teasdale (1998, p. 1) as 'influencing those who have power on behalf of those who do not'. Carpenter (1992, p. 11) defines advocacy as: 'assuming some responsibilities for another person who, for one reason or another, is unable to manage the situation effectively for himself'. Carpenter's definition can be used when discussing the disempowerment of mental health patients such as dementia sufferers. Teasdale (1998, p. 1) describes patients who require advocacy as 'vulnerable and powerless'.

Bandman & Bandman (1990) described the role of the advocate as the protector of a client against abuse, and to safeguard the client's rights. Given that the demented patient is very vulnerable, they are open to abuse and require the strong support of an advocate to ensure their rights are maintained.

Bayne et al (1998, p. 73) described the ideal characteristics of an advocate as having, 'empathy, good communication skills, knowledge of mental health issues, strength of character to be able to stand up to professionals and to be on the side of the client at all times'.

Four types of advocacy have been described by Beresford & Croft (1993):

1. *Legal*: The use of lawyers to defend a person's rights.
2. *Professional*: A representative of the person, such as a case manager.
3. *Citizen*: An unprofessional and unpaid advocate who represents the person's interest due to the disability of that person.
4. *Self*: The person speaks for their own rights and interests.

Teasdale (1998, p. 22) also describes *collective advocacy*, and defines this as, 'an organised group of people campaigning for a particular cause'.

Patients such as Mr James will benefit from an advocate, be that a professional (such as a nurse), a lawyer or a family member. Decisions such as whether Mr and Mrs James should share a room, despite the risk of domestic violence can be jointly discussed with the health professionals and the advocate, and a mutual agreement can then be reached. An advocate can explain all the implications to Mr and Mrs James so that an informed decision can be reached. The advocate can also ensure the total needs and concerns of the extended family are discussed with the social workers and the matron.

References

American Psychiatric Association (1994). DSM-IV: Diagnostic and statistical manual of mental disorders. (4th ed.). Washington: American Psychiatric Association. Cited in: Keady, J. (1999). Dementia. Elderly Care 11(1): 21–26.

Bandman, E.L., Bandman, B. (1990). Nursing ethics through the life span. Englewood Cliffs: Prentice-Hall.

Bayne, R., Nicolson, P., Horton, I. (1998). Counselling and Communication Skills for Medical and Health Practitioners. Leicester: The British Psychological Society Books.

Beresford, P., Croft, S. (1993). Citizen Involvement: A Practical Guide for Change. Basingstoke: Macmillan.

Carpenter, D. (1992). Advocacy. Nursing Times 88(27): 11.

Department of Health (1989). Homes Are For Living In. London: DOH.

Eliopoulos, C. (1993). Gerontological nursing. (3rd ed.). Philadelphia: J.B. Lippincott Company.

Hopker, S. (1999). Drug Treatments and Dementia. London: Jessica Kingsley Publishers.

Iliffe, S., Patterson, L., Gould, M. (1998). Health Care for Older People. London: BMJ Books.

Keady, J., Williams, K. (1998). Counselling skills for carers and early stage dementia care. Elderly Care 10(2): 15–17.

McMahon, C., Isaacs, R. (1997). Care of the Older Person. Oxford: Blackwell Science.

Teasdale, K. (1998). Advocacy in Health Care. Oxford: Blackwell Science.

Wilcock, G. (1999). Living with Alzheimer's Disease and Similar Conditions: A Guide for Families and Carers. (2nd ed.). London: Penguin.

World Health Organisation (1993). The ICD-10 Classification of Mental and Behavioural Disorders: Diagnostic Criteria for Research. Geneva: World Health Organisation. Cited in: Keady, J. (1999). Dementia. Elderly Care 11(1): 21–26.

Dementia: person-centred care: loneliness

Chris Buswell

Molly Fizpatrick is a 78-year-old widow. Her husband, Frank, a former ship builder, died of lung cancer 3 years ago. Molly lived on her own for 6 months in their bungalow. However her son, Sean, noticed that she was not caring for herself as well as everyone thought. He observed that his mother had lost a bit of weight and did not eat any of the meals that his wife, Mary, took round. Having been a housewife all her life, Molly had always been house proud, but Sean witnessed a gradual decline in the standard of housework in the bungalow. Molly agreed with her son that she should go and live with him in their spare bedroom. Molly was glad of this as she had felt lonely since Frank's death and looked forward to spending more time with her grandson and granddaughter.

It took Molly several weeks to get used to the idea of living with her son, his wife and their children. However, she did gain weight and appeared to be her normal happy self. Mary thought Molly a little 'strange' at times. She witnessed Molly doing unusual things, such as putting the alarm clock in the fridge and hanging newspapers on the washing line. Mary put these things down to 'old age', but decided that it was time to tell Sean of her concerns when she witnessed Molly urinating in the lounge metal waste paper bin which she 'mistook' for the lavatory.

Sean reported their concerns to Molly's GP. After several visits to him and a psycho-geriatrician, Molly was diagnosed as being in the early stages of dementia.

Molly, who still had enough insight to realise what was happening to her, was very upset, as was Sean. Both drew on the support of Elizabeth, the district nurse, who came to dress Molly's leg ulcers once a week.

One day Sean asked Elizabeth to stay for a cup of tea and a chat whilst Mary and Molly went into the garden. He said:

'I'm worried about Mum. She seems so sad and lonely, even though she's surrounded by my family. I think she worries a lot too, because some of her friends had dementia and ended up in a nursing home. Mum went to visit one of them and she didn't even recognise Mum. Mum was very shocked. I think she told me this because she worries about losing her marbles, and her memory. I know that Mum isn't too affected by dementia at the moment, but in time we all know that she will get worse. What can I do for her, Elizabeth?'

Question one: Describe loneliness in the elderly and explain why Molly is suffering from it.

15 minutes

Question two: Define person-centred care and outline its relevance for patients with dementia and their families.

15 minutes

Question three: Outline the importance of memories in relation to patients with dementia and give examples of the value this has to their family and friends.

20 minutes

Time allowance: **50 minutes**

Answer to question one:
Describe loneliness in the elderly and explain why Molly is suffering from it.

Before discussing loneliness in the elderly, it may be beneficial to define loneliness. One author described loneliness as an unpleasant condition where an individual feels apart from others (Copel, 1988). It arises from a lack of human intimacy, and can even occur when in the presence of others (Shearer & Davidhizar, 1999).

Eliopoulos (1993, p. 41) states that loneliness 'emphasises all the misfortunes of people who are growing old'. She further explains that other people may avoid elderly people because it reminds them that they themselves will be old one day and they find it difficult to accept the changes that they witness in an older person. Shearer & Davidhizar (1999) argue that the need for human interaction becomes more intense for the elderly as losses and situational stress increase.

Reduced mobility may cause elderly people to become house bound. Some may fear going outside, especially in busy urban areas.

Communication problems such as deafness may hinder conversation and promote feelings of loneliness.

Patients with an altered body image due to disability or continence problems may be afraid to seek outside contact due to the way they perceive themselves to look or smell.

Loneliness should not be mistaken for solitude. Seeking solitude is common for anyone of any age. The elderly may seek periods of solitude so that they can reflect on their life, or reminisce (Eliopoulos, 1993). Some people may prefer a life of solitude and not wish for contact, or they may desire very little contact with others and not feel lonely. Molly may see her son, daughter-in-law and grandchildren every day, but even with loved ones around a person can still feel lonely (Shearer & Davidhizar, 1993).

Elderly patients are much more likely to face the deaths of their fellows than younger people (Lavigne-Pley & Levesque, 1992). As their circle of friends diminishes, elderly people may be left thinking of their own mortality. This may increase their feelings of loneliness as they grieve for dead friends and loved ones (Buswell, 1998).

In Molly's case, she may be feeling lonely after the death of her husband Frank; in fact she may still be grieving for him. She may even be grieving for her loss of independence and the familiar furniture in her bungalow. Although family members such as Molly's son and his wife will be able to make her new surroundings as homely as possible by transferring personal belongings and perhaps favourite pieces of furniture, it will not feel like home for quite a while.

Many older people look forward to visitors, such as the district nurse, coming to see them at home. Some may like the physical contact of a nurse changing dressings, but for others, it may be their only visit, or touch from another person, for a long period of time.

Answer to question two:
Define person-centred care and outline its relevance for patients with dementia and their families.

Person-centred care has been developed by the work of the late Professor Tom Kitwood and the Bradford Dementia Group since the 1980s (Kitwood, 1997a). Kitwood encourages health care professionals to look beyond the behaviour of the person with dementia and to try to understand their behaviour as a form of communication. Rather than seeing the dementia, he suggests that we should be seeing the person underneath the dementia.

Innes & Jacques (1998, p. 17) describe this change in emphasis as being 'from managing behaviour to understanding first and foremost the person and the behaviour in which the person is engaged'. Luckhurst & Ray (1999, p. 30) ask the nurse to, 'look for the potential and abilities of the individual rather than the difficulties and disabilities'.

Kitwood (1997a) also developed the term 'holding'; this is the care needed to keep a person with dementia in a state of well-being so that they feel a sense of purpose and develop high self-esteem.

Kitwood (1997a) developed dementia care mapping to form an empathic view of how patients may experience care and its interactions, and how it will affect their well-being.

In the early stages of dementia, such as in Molly's case, the person may be aware of their memory and behavioural losses (Kitwood, 1997b). The nurse has to respond sensitively and effectively to the individual needs of patients and their loved ones, which may affect the patients' fears for their future (Keady & Williams, 1998).

Answer to question one:
Describe sleep in the older person, and natural changes that occur in old age.

As a person ages there are normal and natural changes to sleep patterns. Older people experience a reduction, or absence, of stage four (also called slow-wave) sleep (Fillit & Picariello, 1998; Eliopoulos, 1993; Tortora & Grabowski, 1996; Howcroft & Jones, 1999). See Box 15.1 for a description of the stages of sleep. There is an increase in nocturnal wakefulness (Fillit & Picariello, 1998; Howcroft & Jones, 1999). Older people find it more difficult to fall asleep (Pascal & Woodhouse, 1994) and are more easily awakened from sleep (Fillit & Picariello, 1998; Howcroft & Jones, 1999). These may lead to the elderly person feeling tired and having periods of sleep during the day. The lack of nocturnal sleep may cause the elderly person to feel irritable and depressed. Eliopoulos (1993) described emotional dysfunction as being caused by lack of REM sleep.

As an elderly person ages, the length of time spent sleeping decreases (Tortora & Grabowski, 1996). An interesting point made by McMahon & Isaacs (1997) is that although the older person needs less sleep time, their time spent in bed may be longer. Could this be because the patient does not accept that less sleep is needed, but still routinely goes to bed at the normal time? Or could it be due to ritualistic care for those elderly people in establishments such as nursing homes, where patients are assisted to bed at times that suit the care provider and not the patient?

Box 15.1 Stages of sleep

Stage 1: This is the transition period between wakefulness and sleep. It generally lasts up to 7 minutes. The person is relaxing with their eyes closed and has fleeting thoughts.

Stage 2: This is the first true stage of sleep. The person is described as just asleep, but it is difficult to awaken them. Dreams may be experienced and the person's eyes may slowly roll from side to side.

Stage 3: This is the first period of moderate deep sleep. The person is very relaxed. Blood pressure and body temperature fall. Muscles are relaxed. It is difficult to awaken the person. This stage occurs approximately 20 minutes after the person falls asleep.

Stage 4: Deep sleep occurs in this stage. It is very difficult to awaken someone in this stage of sleep. The person is very relaxed and if awakened the person responds very slowly. All the person's body functions are reduced.

REM sleep: During rapid eye movement (REM) sleep, most dreaming occurs. After REM sleep the person descends to stages 3 and 4 of non-REM sleep. REM and non-REM sleep alternate throughout the night at approximately 90-minute intervals between REM periods. Sedatives will decrease REM sleep. In the elderly, REM sleep decreases with age.

Adapted from Tortora & Grabowski, 1996

In addition to the normal ageing process's effects on sleep, the elderly person may also be affected by sleep disorders such as narcolepsy or sleep apnoea. It has been estimated that 20–30% of people in their 70s verbalise sleep disturbances (Fillit & Picariello, 1998). These sleep disturbances could be caused by pain, nocturia, emotional traumas resulting from bereavement, or mental health problems such as depression.

Answer to question two:
Identify changes in sleep that can occur in patients with dementia.

Patients with dementia may still be affected by the same natural changes of sleep due to the ageing process. However, the condition of dementia brings with it other problems that will affect the person's sleep pattern and quality of sleep. It has been estimated that approximately 25% of people with dementia have difficulties with sleep (Hopker, 1999).

In dementia there is a progressive degeneration of cortical and subcortical neurones. Howcroft & Jones (1999) argue that this neurological damage extends to the brain structure involved in the sleep/wake functions, and leads to the associated sleep disruption in dementia.

Dementia patients often become confused or agitated in the afternoon or early evening. This is known as 'sundowning' because of the relationship with the setting sun (Howcroft & Jones, 1999; Eliopoulos, 1993). Symptoms can be reduced by ensuring that artificial lighting is switched on before natural light disappears and that night lighting is used. Night lighting can also reduce disorientation caused by dementia patients awakening at night into what they see as an unfamiliar and strange environment. Such feelings can cause the patient to wander, perhaps looking for a more familiar environment, or more familiar objects (Cantes & Rigby, 1997).

Howcroft & Jones (1999) describe that carers of people with dementia often choose care in institutions for their relatives because of disruptive nocturnal behaviour. However it should also be noted that an admission to a nursing home can increase disruptive sleep behaviour.

It can be common for patients with dementia to be prescribed antipsychotic medication by a GP during behavioural disturbances, and for the patient to remain taking such drugs, even if no longer needed (Hopker, 1999). This may have happened to George. His Melleril may have been prescribed following his wife's death, and several months later he may still be following his doctor's advice. Patients with dementia should have their medication regimen routinely assessed by their doctor for effectiveness in controlling symptoms and for possible side-effects. One side-effect of antipsychotic medication is sedation. However, due to this side-effect, antipsychotics may be prescribed in cases of severe agitation (Hopker, 1999). The sedative effect of Melleril will have affected George since he was not agitated when taking them at lunchtime. This would have caused him to sleep in the afternoon, and his subsequent awakening in the early hours of the morning with wandering behaviour.

Answer to question three:
Outline possible alternatives to medication that can help induce a natural sleep in an older person.

Before prescribing any treatment – either natural remedies, changes in lifestyle or drug intervention – the health care professional must first assess the older person's sleep habits. Emphasis must be placed on the normal ageing process changes that will affect an older person's quality and quantity of sleep. It must be assessed whether there are unrealistic expectations, such as retiring at 9.00 p.m. and expecting to sleep peacefully until 8.00 a.m. (Eliopoulos, 1993; Hopker, 1999). An elderly person may need assurance that reduced sleep is normal for an ageing person (Fillit & Picariello, 1998).

During the assessment the health care professional should look for factors that may cause insomnia, such as pain or urinary problems. Patients who are kept awake, or are awakened by pain may find it beneficial to take prescribed analgesics prior to bedtime.

The elderly person should be advised to avoid nicotine, alcohol and drinks with caffeine, such as tea or coffee, before bedtime (Howcroft & Jones, 1999). Caffeine and nicotine contain stimulants that will hinder natural sleep. Hot, milky drinks that relax and aid the inducement of sleep can replace such drinks (Fillit & Picariello, 1998; McMahon & Isaacs, 1997).

Maintaining a regular bedtime and pattern of activity may help the elderly person to reach sleep (Hopker, 1999; McMahon & Isaacs, 1997). A service that may benefit elderly people living at home is the 'tuck-up' or 'twilight' service provided by the community nursing and care team. After an individualised assessment the patient can agree with the nurses or carers as to what time they will come to the patient's home to help them to bed. Thus a patient's regular time for going to bed is maintained, and a sense of normalcy continues.

Some elderly people, particularly those with dementia, may find it beneficial to sleep with subdued lighting (Eliopoulos, 1993).

Within the confines of physical ability, elderly people should be kept active, physically and mentally during the day (Eliopoulos, 1993; McMahon & Issacs, 1997). This prevents daytime napping and promotes sleep at night.

A massage or a warm bath may be of benefit prior to sleep, especially for patients with chronic pain, due to the muscle-relaxing effect these have (Eliopoulos, 1993).

Consideration should be given to the environment to ensure the room is warm and that the person has enough blankets or a high togged quilt. Some elderly people like electric blankets and hot water bottles. Care should be taken when using these since the elderly person will have a reduced response to heat on their skin. This is caused by a reduction of sensory nerve impulses on the skin and the sluggish response of messages sent to the cerebral cortex and hypothalamus.

The mattress of the elderly person should be free of impediments and their pillow(s) supportive (Fillit & Picariello, 1998).

References

Cantes, S., Rigby, P. (1997). Freedom to wander safely. Elderly Care 9(4): 8–10.

Eliopoulos, C. (1993). Gerontological Nursing. (3rd ed.). Philadelphia: J.B. Lippincott Company.

Fillit, H., Picariello, G. (1998). Practical Geriatric Assessment. London: Greenwich Medical Media Ltd.

Hopker, S. (1999). Drug Treatments and Dementia. London: Jessica Kingsley Publishers.

Howcroft, D., Jones, R. (1999). Sleep, older people and dementia. Nursing Times 95(33): 54–56.

McMahon, C., Isaacs, R. (1997). Care of the Older Person: A Handbook for Care Assistants. Oxford: Blackwell Science.

Pascal, J., Woodhouse, K. (1994). The effective management of insomnia. Geriatric Medicine February: 41–44. Cited in: McMahon, C., Isaacs, R. (1997). Care of the Older Person: A Handbook for Care Assistants. Oxford: Blackwell Science.

Tortora, G., Grabowski, S. (1996). Principles of Anatomy and Physiology. (8th ed.). New York: Harper Collins College Publishers.

Diabetes

Vivienne Mathews

> Mr James Walford, a widower, aged 76, is a retired turf accountant. He lives with his daughter and two granddaughters in a bungalow in the suburbs of a large cathedral city. His wife died from breast cancer 10 years ago and he has found it very difficult to adjust to life without her.
>
> Although retired, he has a very busy life, mainly looking after his granddaughters while his daughter is at work. He plays indoor and outdoor bowls, goes swimming on a regular basis and enjoys reading crime and science fiction novels.
>
> Mr Walford is overweight, with type 2 diabetes (non-insulin dependent diabetes), which he has had for 14 years. He feels he habitually overeats, but cannot break his eating pattern of snacking whilst watching television. The understanding he has of his diet, in relation to his diabetes, is poor, as his late wife undertook all the catering arrangements and now his daughter shops and cooks for him, as well as her family.

Question one: What should the main nutritional recommendations be for Mr Walford to enable him to control his diabetes?

10 minutes

Question two: What are the consequences of Mr Walford's poor diet likely to be?

10 minutes

Question three: What aspects of Mr Walford's lifestyle reinforce the tendency to overeat and how can these be counteracted?

10 minutes

Time allowance: **30 minutes**

Answer to question one:
What should the main nutritional recommendations be for Mr Walford to enable him to control his diabetes?

The nutritional recommendations in the management of diabetes include:

- Eating regular meals
- Aiming to eat a balanced diet with decreased amounts of sweetened soft drinks, chocolate, biscuits, cakes and sweets.
- Cutting down on fats but ensuring the fat that is eaten is monosaturated or polyunsaturated
- Eating more high-fibre foods
- Aiming for five portions of vegetables and fruit per day
- Eating more carbohydrate foods
- Not buying special 'diabetic' brands of squash, jams, sweets or biscuits
- Trying to limit the amount of salt eaten
- Taking only moderate amounts of alcohol.

(Adapted from Parkin, 1997)

By following the guidelines mentioned earlier, Mr Walford should be able to improve his glycaemic control and lower lipid levels will ensue (Parkin, 1997).

Answer to question two:
What are the consequences of Mr Walford's poor diet likely to be?

The role of dietary control is to:

- Achieve the most favourable glycaemic control
- Reduce the incidence of hyper- and hypoglycaemia
- Achieve and maintain appropriate weight for height (McGill, 1997)
- Reduce the incidence of diabetic complications, such as cardiovascular disorders.

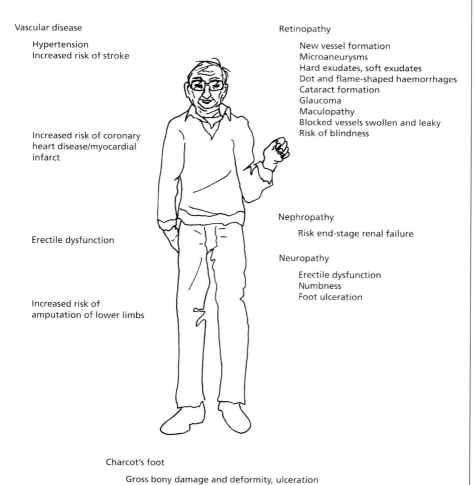

Vascular disease

    Hypertension
    Increased risk of stroke

    Increased risk of coronary
    heart disease/myocardial
    infarct

Erectile dysfunction

    Increased risk of
    amputation of lower limbs

Retinopathy

    New vessel formation
    Microaneurysms
    Hard exudates, soft exudates
    Dot and flame-shaped haemorrhages
    Cataract formation
    Glaucoma
    Maculopathy
    Blocked vessels swollen and leaky
    Risk of blindness

Nephropathy

    Risk end-stage renal failure

Neuropathy

    Erectile dysfunction
    Numbness
    Foot ulceration

    Charcot's foot
        Gross bony damage and deformity, ulceration

Figure 16.1: Chronic complications associated with diabetes.

Mr Walford, as well as other diabetic patients, require advice about their diets, regardless of their treatments, to help them manage stable blood glucose levels, minimise the risk of complications and assist with weight management (Anderson & Genthner, 1990).

By following the dietary recommendations as in answer one, James should have improved glycaemic control, improved lipid levels, decreased complications and be able to achieve some weight loss (British Diabetic Association, 1992).

Answer to question three:
What aspects of Mr Walford's lifestyle reinforces the tendency to overeat and can these be counteracted?

Patients' concerns about their diet are very different from those of the nurse and unless they are taken into account no real patient education can result. There will be frustration, both on the part of the nurse, who labels the patient as 'non-compliant' or a 'failure', and on the part of the patient, who feels his needs are not being met.

Mr Walford must be listened to and lifestyle issues, such as 'Can I eat fish and chips after bowls on a Friday?' or 'What about birthday cake when my granddaughters have their birthdays?', must be addressed.

If the patient becomes demotivated about his illness and the dietary requirements necessary, he will seek advice elsewhere, which may be conflicting, inaccurate or downright dangerous.

Mr Walford and his daughter have a knowledge deficit about the management of his diabetic diet, which should be dealt with as a matter of urgency. Misconceptions about food and why a slightly more specialised diet is needed, a whole range of anxieties and concerns about health, weight and the disease process will influence eating habits, and will, possibly, set the scene for discussions to improve motivation and knowledge.

Once a rapport with Mr Walford has been established, problems with the diet, e.g. his snacking habits, can be explored and clarified. Eating habits are the result of emotional and social situations, such as living with a young family and his beliefs about food and diet that have influenced him in the past. Discussions about what triggers his snacking behaviour, even though he knows it is harmful, and on how to avoid pitfalls and have healthy snacks available are vital. Mr Walford has made mistakes in the past, which he should be encouraged to learn from.

Several studies have shown that the number of abnormal attitudes about food in people with diabetes is high (Durrant, 1997). Emotions have a major role to play in establishing eating habits, so the next step for Mr Walford will be to identify what self-care mechanisms he will be willing to adhere to. If Mr Walford suggests a change in eating habits for himself, he is more likely to follow it through and to understand the responsibility for this solution, and ultimate control of his diabetes, lies with him.

Advice from the nurse can sometimes have a negative effect, by lowering self-esteem and making Mr Walford resistant to change (Travis, 1997).

References

Anderson, R.M., Genthner, R.W. (1990). A guide for assessing a patient's level of personal responsibility for diabetes management. Patient Education and Counselling 16: 269–279.

British Diabetic Association (1992). Dietary recommendations for people with diabetes: an update for the 1990's. Diabetic Medicine 9: 189–202.

Durrant, S. (1997). Psychology and diet. Practical Diabetes International 14(1): 17–19.

McGill, E. (1997). Nutrition and diabetes. Nutrition in practice supplement. No.8. Nursing Times 93(51): 1–6.

Parkin, T. (1997). Patient control in dietary management. Professional Nurse Study Supplement 13(3): S7–S10.

Travis, T. (1997). Patient perceptions of factors that affect adherence to dietary regimens for diabetes mellitus. Diabetes Educator 23(2): 152–156.

Further reading

Brown, F., Cradock, S., Parkin, T. (1997). Diabetes. Professional Nurse Study Supplement 13(3): S2–S15.

Domestic violence

Vivienne Mathews

> Sandra Kingdom is a 33-year-old married woman who lives in a large detached house on a new housing estate. She has two sons, aged 4 and 6, who are looked after during the day by Sandra's grandmother. Sandra and her mother work together, co-owning a small printing firm situated in the city centre.
>
> Sandra's husband, David, is a 47-year-old chief executive of a city banking house. He works in London, commuting daily from his home to his office, and often returning home after 10 p.m. at night. Sandra is expected to entertain his clients at short notice and to attend office functions in the city, which, increasingly, she finds difficult to do owing to the constraints of her own business and a young family.
>
> Sandra and David both admit that their marriage is not a comfortable one, mainly because of David's short temper and inclination to sulk and Sandra's difficulty in juggling her domestic duties with her social and business life. She admits to being ill at ease whilst entertaining, which is very apparent in her tense, uneasy manner and her awkwardness in talking to strangers.
>
> Sandra was admitted to the Accident & Emergency department of the local general hospital at noon on a Sunday in May. She had multiple injuries, especially around her head, neck, face and breasts, which were attributed to a fall downstairs whilst slightly tipsy.
>
> David accompanied her to the hospital, but left abruptly, saying he had a headache and two small boys to look after.

Question one: Give a definition of domestic violence and comment on its prevalence in the UK.

15 minutes

Question two: How can victims of domestic violence be recognised?

10 minutes

Question three: What can be done to improve practice in the recognition of domestic violence?

15 minutes

Time allowance: **40 minutes**

Answer to question one:
Give a definition of domestic violence and comment on its prevalence in the UK.

Domestic violence covers a broad area of abuse and neglect, but can be seen as a pattern of inappropriate brutal, coercive control by one person over another (Schechter, 1987). It frequently describes physical abuse but psychological abuse, which is more covert, can be included as it takes the form of threats and verbal abuse.

Exploitation can consist of compelling a person to act against their wishes, as in forcing a person to take part in deviant sex acts, or in preventing them from making choices that all people should be free to make, e.g. when to go to bed, what to eat or drink or wear, when to smoke a cigarette or to have a bath (Baumhover & Beall, 1996).

> **NB:** Exploitation is the term used to refer to an act that manipulates a person or their goods, property or money to the disadvantage of that person, but to the advantage of the exploiter.
>
> (Baumhover & Beall, 1996)

Domestic violence is seen as a problem mainly for women and is the direct result of the second-class standing women have within marriage and society as a whole (Davidson, 1997). Domestic violence, contrary to most public opinions, is not confined to unstable or dysfunctional marriages; it is prevalent in all classes of society, in all age groups, occupations, racial and religious groups. Research has shown that at least one in five marriages is likely to involve some form of domestic violence (Victim Support, 1992).

Andrews & Brown (1988) report that 22–35% of women visiting Accident & Emergency departments attend for injuries caused by domestic violence, or 'battery' as it is commonly known.

Sometimes a nurse's understanding of domestic violence will depend upon its personal impact; 20% of nurses will have experienced domestic violence at first hand and may repress their feelings, rationalising their experiences by using personal beliefs and recognised social standards to do so. Nurses who have not experienced domestic violence may reject the patient because of disbelief or powerlessness or emotional withdrawal from the patient, characterised by rejection of the patient.

A full appreciation of all the practical, emotional and social elements that play a part in each relationship, identification of the feelings of worthlessness, frustration and guilt experienced by the victim and recognition of the fear of pursuit and retaliation that underpins the situation should be understood (Davidson, 1997). Nurses are often unwilling to probe, as the idea of the family as private territory, with problems that should be resolved by the family members themselves, persists, and can affect the way domestic violence is seen and responded to by nurses (King & Ryan, 1989).

Answer to question two:
How can victims of domestic violence be recognised?

Nurses should be aware of the more common signs and symptoms of domestic violence, starting with time and privacy to allow the victim to talk about their experiences. This may then be followed by a full physical assessment so that signs of old and new trauma can be recognised. Often the history of the incident and the injuries present do not match up, as in Sandra's, where a fall down the stairs would present with bruising and grazes to the legs and arms, not just the head, neck and breasts. Another indication of possible abuse is that of a time delay in presenting at a hospital for treatment and the actual time of the incident.

Again, as in Sandra's case, the 'accident' happened the evening before but was only reported some 12 hours later.

When David left Sandra, he commented that it was a lot of fuss to make over a small thing, which may be another indication that violence may have occurred, as injuries are often trivialised by one, or both, parties.

There may have been signs of fear, panic or extreme anxiety on Sandra's part whilst she was being questioned and examined, which may be coupled with withdrawal and apprehension, especially in the presence of her husband, and a low level of self-esteem. There may have been repressed anger or expressed antagonism on her part towards her husband who appeared, at first, overattentive and then disengaged completely.

All these signs may indicate that domestic friction has exploded into violence, resulting in the hospitalisation of Sandra.

Answer to question three:
What can be done to improve practice in the recognition and treatment of domestic violence?

As already stated, nurses need to recognise and become familiar with overt and covert signs of domestic violence. It should be remembered that a non-judgemental approach may be the key towards disclosure of intensely private and personal information, but some assurances that the victim will be believed and have a measure of security is of equal importance (Hague & Malos, 1993).

A private, safe environment, with plenty of time to discuss experiences and a possible course of action for the future, is needed.

Box 17.1 lists a number of indicators of physical abuse.

Box 17.1 Indicators of physical abuse

- Human bite marks
- Sprains
- Lacerations
- Bruises
- Dislocations
- Puncture wounds
- Internal injuries
- Dehydration
- Malnutrition
- Imprint bruises (marks in the shape of fingers, belts, sticks etc.)
- Burns (inflicted by cigarettes, ropes, matches, irons, immersion in hot water)
- Marks left by a gag
- Eye injuries (black eye, conjunctivitis (redeye), detatched retina)
- Missing teeth
- Unexplained scars
- Alopecia (spotty balding) from pulling hair.

(Adapted from Baumhover & Beall, 1996)

The victim should be informed that a criminal act has taken place and that they are entitled to police intervention, but as always, the patient must decide for themselves what to do and this decision must be respected (Davidson, 1997).

Keep up-to-date, comprehensive records as these will show other health care professionals that the situation is serious and ongoing. Nursing documentation may be needed in any legal proceedings or housing requests. Regular training and updating should be forthcoming on this issue. Colleagues and other agencies should exchange information and develop guidelines for intervention and referral procedures. The factors that make this a difficult topic should be addressed by enlarging personal knowledge and understanding of domestic violence by reading educational books and journals on the subject.

Information about places of refuge, local support groups, housing department contacts and welfare benefits should be available, with resource lists that may help to resolve some of the practicalities of an emergency situation.

Understanding the nature of domestic violence is not easy, but nurses should be knowledgeable about national and local resources. They should also be open and non-judgemental about the problem, aiming to be skilled in listening and uncovering the existence of possible physical abuse. The nurse should be able to challenge circumstances that undermine the health and dignity of victims of domestic violence.

References

Andrews, B., Brown, G. (1988). Violence in the community; a biographical approach. British Journal of Psychiatry 153: 305–312.

Baumhover, L.A., Beall, S.C. (1996). Abuse, Neglect and Exploitation of Older Patients. London: Jessica Kingsley Publishers.

Davidson, J. (1997). Domestic violence; the nursing response. Professional Nurse 12 (9): 632–634.

Hague, J., Malos, E. (1993). Domestic Violence. Cheltenham: New Clarion Press.

King, M., Ryan, J. (1989). Abused women; dispelling the myths and encouraging intervention. Nurse Practitioner 14: 47–48.

Schechter, S. (1987). Guidelines for mental health professionals in domestic violence cases. In: Davidson, J. (1997). Domestic violence: the nursing response. Professional Nurse 12 (9): 632–634.

Victim Support (1992). Domestic Violence: A Report of a National Inter-agency Working Party. London: Victim Support.

Ethics: compliance

Vivienne Mathews

Mrs Bettina Ormerod is a widow, aged 94. She lives alone in a state of considerable personal neglect. She has no visible carers. It is possible that relatives, who reside in the same village, have refused to have anything to do with her because of her squalid living conditions. Her personal state is filthy and that of the house is decayed, fetid and repulsive. She appears to live in one room, downstairs, where she eats, sleeps and goes to the lavatory in a bucket.

Mrs Ormerod's main diet is tinned macaroni cheese followed by tinned custard. Her edentulous mouth makes chewing very difficult. She has had meals on wheels and home helps in the past, but all of them have been dismissed on one trivial count or another. She refuses all offers of help from 'them busy bodies' at the social services, allowing only a neighbour into her home on a daily basis. Other neighbours eschew her presence and complain, bitterly, about the stench coming from her house.

Mrs Ormerod has chronic bronchitis and heart failure, for which hospital admission has been offered and turned down. She refuses to take her medication, except on a very irregular basis, overdosing and omitting tablets as she pleases. Her compliance with any type of therapeutic regimen, e.g. dosette boxes, is non-existent.

Mrs Ormerod has serious health problems and socially, because of a breakdown in domestic and personal care, has been reduced to living in isolation and hostility.

Question one: What are the ethical dilemmas facing health care professionals in this case?

15 minutes

Question two: Identify reasons why some elderly people do not comply with prescribed medication regimens.

10 minutes

Question three: What can be done to encourage Mrs Ormerod to comply with her medication regimen?

15 minutes

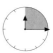

Time allowance: **40 minutes**

Answer to question one:
What are the ethical dilemmas facing health care professionals in this case?

Mrs Ormerod firmly refuses all offers of help. She lives in squalor of her own choosing but that has resulted in her being rejected by relatives and neighbours alike. In view of her increasing age, the situation, by normal standards, is unacceptable.

Mrs Ormerod should be allowed to live as she chooses, ending her life in her own way, but she lives in a village community, in close proximity with her immediate neighbours, who are affected by the stale food, dirt, smell and vermin emanating from her house. Tolerance by the neighbours, who are being offended, daily, is wearing extremely thin, but is there a balance between Mrs Ormerod's personal freedom to do as she pleases and theirs to live a life free of vermin infestation and stench?

Who takes action? The relatives have withdrawn completely or lost interest in trying to help. There may be family feuds and a considerable degree of rancour between them. The GP continues to treat and prescribe, but fails to persuade Mrs Ormerod to comply. If she were to die amid this filth, would he be guilty of medical neglect? If this were the case, her death could be classified as suicide by self-neglect. It may be that Mrs Ormerod is right in her non-compliance in that treatment will not make any difference to her condition. Yet, the law could be invoked in cases where elderly people are considered to be a danger to themselves or others, to place her in hospital or a place of safety.

Many people accept that treatment should be given, or changes 'for the better' be forced on elderly people for 'their own good', but should this be done at the expense of their personal wishes? (Williams, 1989).

> **NB:** If an elderly person cannot manage their affairs because of mental infirmity, an Enduring Power of Attorney may be organised. Power of Attorney enables some other person to sign documents in the name of the donor. It can only be used when the donor is of sound mind, but if their mental capabilities then deteriorate, the existing power becomes invalid and the Enduring Power of Attorney is invoked.
>
> (Williams, 1989)

The law does not cater for people of sound mind who chose to live in normally unacceptable conditions, despite their deteriorating physical condition.

Answer to question two:
Identify reasons why some elderly people do not comply with prescribed medication regimens.

Cargill (1992) has defined non-compliance as the degree to which subjects diverge from a prescribed regimen. There is a lack of adherence to the prescription and/or its instruction for some reason or another.

Rajaei-Dehkordi & MacPherson (1997) claim that there are three categories of non-compliance:

1. *Accidental:* the patient forgets to take the dose or does so incorrectly because of poor understanding.
2. *Triggered:* the patient may feel better, or worse, when taking prescribed medication so stops taking it, or it could be stopped as it is 'doing them no good at all'.
3. *Intentional:* the patient takes a conscious decision not to take medicines as recommended. In this case, there may be complex physical, mental and social factors that will affect their decision-making processes.

Wright (1993) claims that compliance with a medical regimen is approximately 50%, so the incidence of non-compliance is just as high but with attendant problems of cost, time and morbidity.

The reasons why elderly people do not comply with medication include:

- Forgetfulness
- Medicine is unpleasant to take
- Diminished visual acuity
- Decreased physical strength
- Poor coordination
- Choice not to
- Fear of side-effects
- Decreased comprehension
- Unawareness of the importance of medication
- Inadequate labelling
- Inappropriate information given
- Medication changes
- Inconvenience of taking medications
- Inability to swallow tablets prescribed
- Complicated regimen to follow
- Lack of understanding about medication and dosage
- Lack of supervised practice
- Conflicting advice given
- Lack of confidence in person prescribing medication
- Difficulty in following instructions, e.g. not at home when dose is due.

(Adapted from Nyatanga, 1997)

Answer to question three:
What can be done to encourage Mrs Ormerod to comply with her medication regimen?

Non-compliance should not be seen as an act of defiance, as some doctors believe and therefore blame patients for being forgetful, careless and/or 'bloody minded' (Wright, 1993). Neither sex, race, religion, intelligence nor level of general education appears to have a bearing upon compliance (Parker, 1997).

A regimen that is as simple as possible, that is tailor-made for Mrs Ormerod may provide a solution. Taking tablets, all at once, at breakfast time for example, then becomes part of her daily routine.

It should be remembered that not all elderly people can administer their own medications, and therefore, as in Mrs Ormerod's case, an assessment should be made to determine her mental and physical abilities, as well as her willingness to take responsibility for taking her drugs (Ryan & Jacques, 1997).

Coercion is not recommended, but gentle persuasion, assistance with any difficulties that may arise, better communication and patient education will allow patients to take an active part in decision making about their future (Moir, 1996).

It has been reported by Parker (1997) that elderly people who are satisfied with levels of communication are more likely to follow advice. Importantly, a further factor in non-compliance is how much the elderly person can remember of what they are told, so that if follow-up information, in leaflet form, is available, understanding as to why the medication is taken is reinforced in this way. Also, a demonstration on how to take the medication, using plain, clear instructions by a person who has built up a rapport with Mrs Ormerod will help with compliance, as will very clear labelling of containers.

As long as Mrs Ormerod's motivational characteristics are remembered, then she will learn what she needs to know (Ryan & Jacques, 1997).

Compliance may depend on simple factors, such as whether she can actually get hold of a prescription from the GP and then get it filled by a chemist? A home delivery service may be the answer for Mrs Ormerod. Elderly people may have problems opening containers, reading labels, swallowing tablets or capsules or in using inhalers or administrating eye drops, in which case, each difficulty should be considered in turn and dealt with.

Memory aids, such as medication record cards or compliance devices can be made available for her.

The nurse is often best placed to be the patient's advocate, to achieve a balance between daily life and a medication regimen (Marland, 1998). The community nurse, in collaboration with Mrs Ormerod, could negotiate a suitable, easy-to-take medication system. She could encourage Mrs Ormerod to take an active part in decision making and reassure her if she is anxious over side-effects or other difficulties she may have.

Non-compliance is a complex issue for Mrs Ormerod, as it can have a negative impact on the care she receives from health care professionals and her physical health. It may leave nurses and doctors feeling powerless and frustrated, but should not induce them to withdraw their support from Mrs Ormerod.

References

Cargill, J.M. (1992). Medication compliance in elderly people: influencing variables and interventions. Journal of Advanced Nursing 17(4): 422–426.

Marland, G. (1998). Partnership encourages patients to comply with treatment. Nursing Times 94 (27): 58–59.

Moir, S.D. (1996). Monitoring Elder Compliance and Response. New York: Churchill Livingstone.

Nyatanga, B. (1997). Psychosocial theories of patient non-compliance. Professional Nurse 12(5): 331–334.

Parker, R. (1997). Self administration of drugs by older people. Professional Nurse 12(5): 328–330.

Rajaei-Dehkordi, Z., MacPherson, G. (1997). Drug-related problems in older people. Nursing Times 93(28): 54–56.

Ryan, A., Jacques, I. (1997). Medication compliance in older people. Elderly Care 9(5): 15–20.

Wright, E.C. (1993). How many aunts has Matilda? Lancet 342(8876): 909–913.

Williams, E.I. (1989). Caring for Elderly People in the Community. (2nd ed.). London: Chapman & Hall Ltd.

Further reading

Fuller, D., Edmondson, H. (1996). Drug regimes: assessing patient compliance. Elderly Care 8(6): 22–24.

Facial disfigurement

Barbara Marjoram

Andrea Goldberg is a slim, petite 17-year-old who is presently taking her school examinations prior to pursuing her chosen career. She has been thinking, for some time, of pursuing a career in tourism. She has lived in Gibraltar and America as her father is in the Navy and she has always enjoyed travelling abroad with her parents on holiday. She will be sitting Spanish and French examinations prior to starting at the local further education college, where she will study tourism.

Andrea lives at home with her parents and elder brother, aged 22, and younger sister, aged 12. She gets on well with her parents, brother and sister and has a small gathering of close friends. As yet she has had no boyfriends. Her only employment so far has been as a paper deliverer for the local newsagent, something at which she has been very capable and efficient for the past 3 years. Her hobbies include reading, especially about foreign countries and computer games. She rarely goes to nightclubs with her friends as she is rather shy about her appearance.

Andrea was born with a 'port wine' birthmark that involves the right side of her face and ear. She is very sensitive about her appearance and has become more withdrawn over the last 5 years as she has developed into a young woman. She cannot remember any time at school when she was not picked on and bullied because of her unusual appearance and was even called 'elephant woman' by some very unsympathetic schoolmates.

Andrea and her parents have decided to ask for professional help for the disfigurement and counselling in the hope that Andrea will become less withdrawn.

Question one: The way individuals view body image is complex and can be classified into four dimensions – perception, cognition, social and aesthetic (Thompson, 1990) – Expand these terms.

Question two: Body image is developed during childhood; how will this affect Andrea in her early adult years?

Question three: Andrea has become quite withdrawn due to the bullying and the need to develop into what she considers a socially acceptable young woman. As Trust (1992 in Trevelyan 1996) identifies, disfigurement, whether acquired or congenital, can 'be as disruptive of normal life as disabling injury'. Who can help Andrea overcome these problems and how?

Time allowance: **20 minutes**

Answer to question one:
The way individuals view body image is complex and can be classified into four dimensions – perception, cognition, social and aesthetic (Thompson, 1990) – Expand these terms.

Perception is the way individuals experience the body, for example how large Andrea feels the port wine stain is. *Cognition* is the way individuals think of the body, for example Andrea may feel that her body does not allow her to carry out her chosen role in life. *Social* is the way individuals feel that the body image is shared between people. Andrea may feel that her image is very important to her and the bullying she experienced is others voicing their opinions of her body image. *Aesthetic* is the feeling that the body is something that is attractive or beautiful. Andrea may feel satisfied or dissatisfied with her appearance (Thompson, 1990).

Answer to question two:
Body image is developed during childhood; how will this affect Andrea in her early adult years?

Body image is developed during the school years and refined during adult years. During this time Andrea will be learning to value her physical appearance, often in gender terms, as well as beginning to manipulate her body's appearance so that she can be fashionably acceptable (Price, 1993).

As Partridge & Robinson (1994, p. 54) highlight, 'frequent exposure to negative social experiences can result in feelings of anxiety, inadequacy and lowered self-esteem, which in turn can lead to social avoidance, isolation and depression'.

Andrea has lived with her disfigurement all of her life and may have experienced feelings of being an outsider, which she may have found acutely painful and psychologically detrimental. Broder & Strauss (1991) identified that 69% of children and young adults with facial disfigurement suffered from psychological problems that increased with age.

Answer to question three:

Andrea has become quite withdrawn due to the bullying and the need to develop into what she considers a socially acceptable young woman. As Trust (1992 in Trevelyan 1996) identifies, disfigurement, whether acquired or congenital, can 'be as disruptive of normal life as disabling injury'. Who can help Andrea overcome these problems and how?

Andrea's family may be in a position to give her support by helping her to appraise her own self-worth, her self-esteem and ways to deal with problems in the future. Any individual with a disfigurement needs specialist education and support. As Trust (1992 in Trevelyan 1996) identifies, disfigurement should be approached as 'a total problem, skin deep, mind deep and societal'.

Andrea should be encouraged to seek advice from the local dermatology department, the British Red Cross and/or a qualified beautician, who can advise her about possible treatment including cosmetic camouflage. The other possible treatment is laser surgery for the port wine stain, but this is a long-term proposition and not all hospitals have these facilities. The charity Changing Faces has also developed workshops that put the emphasis on improving social and communication skills, which is backed up by individual sessions and counselling.

References

Broder, H., Strauss, R. (1991). Psychosocial problems and referrals among oral-facial team patients. Journal of Rehabilitation 57(1): 31–36.

Partridge, J., Robinson, E. (1994). Changing faces: two years on. Nursing Standard May 18: 8(34): 54–58.

Price, B. (1993). Diseases and altered body image in children. Paediatric Nursing 5(6): 18–21.

Thompson, J. (1990). Body Image Disturbance: Assessment and Treatment. Oxford: Pergamon Press.

Trust, D. (1992). Disfigurement: a cover up story? Practice Nursing January: 16. In: Trevelyan, J. (1996). Looking good: wigs and camouflage. Nursing Times Sep 25–Oct 1: 92(39): 44, 46.

Further reading

Carlisle, D. (1991). Face value. Nursing Times October 16: 87(42): 26–28.

Partridge, J. (1991). Staring prejudice in the face. Nursing Times October 16: 87(42): 28–30.

Price, B. (1990). Body Image: Nursing Concepts and Care. London: Prentice Hall.

Useful address

Changing Faces
1 and 2 Junction Mews
London W2 1PN
Tel: 020 7706 4234
E-mail: info@faces.demon.co.uk

Faecal incontinence

Barbara Marjoram

> Mr Paul Noyce, aged 48, is married to Joy and they have two children, aged 7 and 12. He has little time for hobbies and finds that after a day's work he falls asleep in front of the television. His only exercise is when the whole family go swimming on a Saturday afternoon.
>
> Mr Noyce works in the city offices of a large publishing firm. He frequently has to entertain visiting authors and agents. His job is fairly stressful and this has resulted in his being very tense. He often suffers from headaches and painful shoulders, which he contributes to his stressful lifestyle that is 'getting him down'. He often takes analgesics to treat the headaches and painful shoulders. He has experienced episodes of insomnia and occasionally takes sleeping tablets that have been prescribed by his GP.
>
> He sometimes complains of constipation, but for the past 2 weeks he has been experiencing faecal incontinence. This has caused him a great deal of embarrassment as it has been difficult for him to disguise the smell of the expelled faeces.
>
> Mr Noyce has now visited his GP for advice.

Question one: Define faecal incontinence and identify its prevalence.

Question two: Identify five possible causes of Mr Noyce's faecal incontinence.

Question three: What advice should Mr Noyce be given by his GP?

Question four: List and explain five possible causes of Mr Noyce's constipation.

Time allowance: **15 minutes**

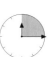

Answer to question one:
Define faecal incontinence and identify its prevalence.

Faecal incontinence is the expulsion of faeces, liquid or gas from the bowel at an undesirable time. It may affect one in 20 people and can occur at any age. (See Useful Websites.)

Answer to question two:
Identify five possible causes of Mr Noyce's faecal incontinence.

- Temporary loss of control caused by diarrhoea
- Disease or injury, for example, permanent or progressive conditions such as cerebrovascular accident, spinal cord damage or multiple sclerosis
- Infection
- Ulcerative colitis or Crohn's disease, which can lead to faecal urge incontinence
- Impacted faeces with overflow
- Stress incontinence caused by chronic straining, trauma or a congenital defect
- Laxative abuse.

(Marjoram 1999: In Hogson & Simpson (Eds) 1999)

(see Useful Websites)

Answer to question three:
What advice should Mr Noyce be given by his GP?

The initial treatment will be to relieve Mr Noyce's constipation and this may be achieved by administering suppositories or an enema every 2–3 days and then instigating a regimen to prevent recurrence.

Mr Noyce will need to be advised to reduce the intake of analgesics as many of these cause constipation. However, without giving advice on reducing stress, this may not be achievable. He will need advice on changing his diet to one that is well balanced and high in fibre (see Floella George profile, p. 37). He will need to increase his fluid intake and be advised to drink 30–35 ml/kg body weight/day but avoid excess alcohol and caffeine as these act as diuretics. He should be advised to take advantage of the body's normal gastrocolic reflex by attending to elimination needs after a meal. Mr Noyce should also be encouraged to increase his exercise level as exercise encourages the motility of the gastrointestinal tract. Although Mr Noyce may use laxatives, these should only be used as a short-term measure as prolonged use may result in dependency (Marjoram, 1999 In: Hogston & Simpson (Eds) 1999).

Answer to question four:
List and explain five possible causes of Mr Noyce's constipation.

- Drugs: tranquillisers, narcotics, anticholinergics, some analgesics (especially those containing codeine) and antacids containing aluminium, which reduce the motility of the gastrointestinal tract
- Disease: obstruction external or internal to the intestines, for example an abdominal tumour. Other causes are irritable bowel syndrome, diverticular disease and neurological deficiencies
- Psychiatric conditions: depression
- Diet: low in fibre or inadequate food intake
- Lack of fluid: insufficient fluid intake or excess alcohol and/or caffeine causes diuresis
- Immobility: decreased mobility reduces motility of the gastrointestinal tract
- Painful defecation: from anal fissure or haemorrhoids (Marjoram, 1999. In: Hogston & Simpson, 1999).

Reference

Marjoram, B. (1999). Elimination. In: Hogston, R., Simpson, P.M. (Eds) Foundations of Nursing Practice. Basingstoke: Macmillan: 143–144.

Further reading

Addison, R. (1996). Treating faecal incontinence. Community Nurse 2(10): 32.
Chelvanayagam, S., Norton, C. (1999). Causes and assessment of faecal incontinence. British Journal of Community Nursing 4(1): 28–35.
Kamm, M. Faecal incontinence. British Medical Journal 316(7130): 528–532.

Useful Websites

Aetiology of faecal incontinence (http://www.bdf.org.uk/leaflets/bowelcon.html [Accessed 1999, July 14])
Maintaining bowel control (http://www.dpa.org.sg/sfcs/wong2.html [Accessed 1999, July 14])

Glaucoma

Vivienne Mathews

William Cameron is 72 years old and enjoys retirement with his wife, Ruth. They live in a comfortable detached house, in a quiet city suburb. William goes to the local leisure centre once or twice a week for a swim and a game of table tennis, while Ruth walks the dog and gardens when the weather permits.

They are both in good health; William has a 'touch' of arthritis and Ruth had a hysterectomy 18 years ago. They eat a balanced diet, do not smoke and both take some exercise on a weekly basis.

One morning, on his return from the leisure centre William complained that he felt 'a bit odd'; his head felt woolly and, unusually, he had no appetite for his lunch.

Ruth insisted that he visit the doctor, where he revealed that he had noticed 'halos' around any lights that were on, had a nagging headache and had difficulty reading the paper.

William was diagnosed as having acute glaucoma, with an intraocular pressure of 80 mmHg.

NB: The normal range for intraocular pressure is between 12–21 mmHg.

(Beed,1992)

Question one: Label the diagram of the eye in Figure 21.1 and give a definition of acute glaucoma.

10 minutes

Question two: What are the most common causes of glaucoma and how is the eye affected by this condition?

10 minutes

Question three: Outline the treatment available for William's glaucoma.
10 minutes

Question four: How can William and his wife adapt their lifestyle to cope with this condition?

10 minutes

Time allowance: **40 minutes**

Answer to question one:

Label the diagram of the eye in Figure 21.1 and give a definition of acute glaucoma.

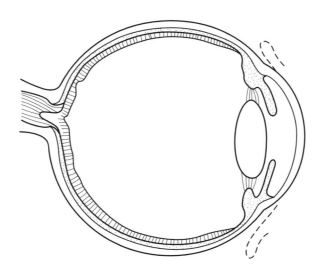

Figure 21.1: Diagram of the eye.

Two definitions of glaucoma include:

1. Glaucoma is an abnormal elevation of intraocular pressure of sufficient duration to cause damage to the eye and changes in visual function (Perry & Tullo,1990).

2. Glaucoma is an increased intraocular pressure due to obstruction to the outflow of aqueous from the eye, caused by: (a) inflammation, (b) congenital abnormality, (c) a narrow angle at the root of the iris in long-sighted eyes, (d) unknown origin (chronic simple glaucoma) (Oxford Concise Medical Dictionary, 1994).

NB: Check the accuracy of your labelling in a nationally recognised anatomy and physiology book such as: Rutishauser S. *Physiology and Anatomy: A Basis for Nursing and Health Care*. Edinburgh: Churchill Livingstone 1996).

Answer to question two:
What are the common causes of glaucoma and how is the eye affected by this condition?

The maintenance of a balance between aqueous humor production and its drainage supports pressure within the eye (intraocular pressure), which helps to maintain the shape of the eyeball. Pressure varies throughout the day, being higher in the morning than during the night (Beed, 1992).

Acute-angle closure glaucoma is not common and is usually present in one eye only. Aqueous humor is prevented from leaving the eye by the drainage angle of the anterior chamber being shut off, which then causes intense pressure to build up within the eye. Unless the pressure is relieved immediately, permanent damage to the eye will occur (International Glaucoma Association, 1989).

This condition often occurs in elderly people, in whom the lens becomes enlarged through the ageing process. In this state, the iris and cornea are much closer than normal, and as the aqueous humor persistently flows through the narrow spaces between these structures, the gap narrows and/or closes so that the aqueous humor cannot pass through the pupil to drain away. Pressure accumulates behind the iris, forcing it forward and into contact with the cornea. In consequence, the intraocular pressure may rise to 70 mmHg (Beed, 1992).

The signs and symptoms of glaucoma include:
- Intense pain in the eye
- Nausea and vomiting
- Visual disturbances
- 'Halos' around lights
- Generalised headaches.

NB: Acute glaucoma is more common in men than in women, and can be effectively treated if detected early.

Answer to question three:
Outline the treatment available for William's glaucoma.

The pressure in the eye must be lowered to a safe level, either by decreasing the amount of aqueous humor secreted or by increasing the outflow from the eye.
 Both these actions can be achieved by oral medication and eye drops:

The following is true regarding use of *eye drops*:
- Used more commonly for chronic open-angle glaucoma
- Can be effective
- Used several times a day for life
- Regular reviews at eye clinics are needed
- Education on how to instil drops properly is required.

Oral medication can also decrease secretions. There are four groups of drugs used to treat glaucoma:

1. Miotics: This class of drug works by making the ciliary muscle of the eye contract, which will cause an increase in the flow of aqueous humor through tension on the trabecular meshwork of the eye (Beed, 1992). A serious side-effect of this drug means that the pupil remains constricted, which is the desired action in acute glaucoma, but may cause visual problems in elderly people.

2. Beta-blockers: This drug will reduce the production of aqueous humor by blocking beta adrenoreceptors in the heart and lungs, so lowering intra-ocular pressure. The major side-effect of this type of medication is bradycardia and respiratory distress, which will occur even when given topically. Beta-blockers can also cause lethargy and shortness of breath, which may not in initial stages be associated with the use of eye drops. This is especially true in elderly people who may think that their increased tiredness is due to the effects of old age. A more selective beta-blocker eye drop is now available that may lessen these symptoms (Winfield, 1991).

3. Adrenaline: This drug is used when all other actions have been unsuccessful. Adrenaline may be responsible for reducing the production of aqueous humor and for increasing outflow. Because of its effect on the heart, adrenaline should be used cautiously in elderly people with hypertension or heart disease. It may cause the eye to redden and sting on instillation (Beed, 1992).

4. Carbon anhydrase inhibitors: This drug is used when a rapid decrease in intraocular pressure is required, such as in acute glaucoma. It can be given orally or by i.v. infusion. It is a diuretic and can cause an electrolyte imbalance, tingling in the fingers and toes, loss of appetite, drowsiness, depression and rashes (Beed, 1992).

NB: A recent advance in the treatment of glaucoma is the use of a holmium laser, which will make a drainage hole through the sclera into the anterior chamber of the eye. This can be performed in a day surgery situation.

(Kennedy, 1992)

Answer to question four:
How can William and his wife adapt their lifestyle to cope with this condition?

Explanation

Explanations of the disease and the treatment options open to them will have to be clearly outlined and any questions answered as frankly and fully as possible.

Written material

This should be given to back up the verbal information given (Oliver, 1993). Several pharmaceutical companies produce booklets and diagrams free of charge.

Condition

It is important that William and Ruth realise that this is a lifelong condition and eye drops will always need to be used, unless surgery is an option open to them.

Treatment

Some miotic-type drugs, such as pilocarpine, will sting on instillation. It may be that William will have to become used to waiting a few minutes, following the use of eye drops, to allow the eye to return to 'normal'. The eye drops must be used four times per day.

Good technique should be taught for instilling eye drops. Both William and Ruth should be instructed on the correct procedure. Self-administration is the best goal, but over a long period, another person competent in this task may reduce the effort of this undertaking.

Compliance

Regular attendance at the eye clinic is important, as vision may be lost without proper care and treatment. Reassurance should be given that, with proper medical supervision, it is unlikely that vision will deteriorate significantly.

There is an association (the International Glaucoma Association) for people with glaucoma, which provides support and information; it also seeks to raise public awareness of glaucoma and the research that is being carried out for its prevention and treatment.

Although there is a high incidence of glaucoma, it is easily detected and treated. Awareness of this condition, how it is diagnosed and the principles of treatment can help reduce the number of people who suffer loss of vision as a result of glaucoma.

References

Beed, P. (1992). Glaucoma: effective care can save sight. Nursing Standard 7(12): 3–8.

International Glaucoma Association (1989). Glaucoma '89: A Guide for Patients. London: King's College Hospital.

Kennedy, S. (1992). Laser filtering: an outpatient procedure? Opthalmology Times 16(1): 1–27.

Oliver, R.W. (1993). Psychology and Health Care. London: Baillière Tindall.

Oxford Concise Medical Dictionary (4th ed.) (1994). Oxford: Oxford University Press.

Perry, J., Tullo, A., (1990). Care of the Opthalmic Patient. London: Chapman & Hall.

Rutishauser, S. (1994). Physiology and Anatomy: A Basis for Nursing and Health Care. Edinburgh: Churchill Livingstone.

Winfield, A.J. (1991). Assisting patients with their eye drops. British Journal of Pharmaceutical Practice 10(12): 14.

Hearing loss: communication

Barbara Marjoram

Agnes Rivendale is a 84-year-old woman who lives in a residential home on the edge of town. She has been living at the home for the past 6 years, since the death of her husband. Agnes has three daughters, six grandchildren and one great granddaughter aged 3 years. One of her daughters visits at least once a week and the family ensure that Agnes is included in all the family gatherings. She has reduced mobility due to rheumatoid arthritis, which has affected her hips and knees. She enjoys playing bingo, scrabble, cards and taking part in the weekly exercise session.

The home often organises visits to the local gardens and in the summer, a visit to the seaside. Until recently, Agnes has always attended the trips to the theatre, which have occurred three times a year, but increasingly has found it frustrating as she cannot follow the plot because of her difficulty in hearing every word.

Over the past few years her daughters have found it increasingly difficult to communicate with their mother, as she appears not to hear them, but when they raise their voices they are 'told off' for shouting. Her eldest daughter has had a word with the matron of the home, who will ask the GP to assess Mrs Rivendale on his next visit.

The GP has now visited Agnes and having examined her ears with an auriscope, has been unable to identify any external reason for her hearing loss, although she has a small amount of cerumen (wax) in her external auditory meatus. The GP arranged for a hearing test at the local hospital, and the results suggest Agnes' hearing loss is due to presbycusis. A post-aural hearing aid has been prescribed for her in the hope that this may improve her communication with her family, friends and staff.

Question one: What is presbycusis and how will it affect Agnes' hearing?

Question two: Identify three other causes of sensorineural deafness.

Question three: Name the other type of hearing loss and identify three causes.

Question four: Explain the care of a hearing aid.

Question five: How could Agnes' ability to hear and understand what is communicated to her be improved?

Time allowance: **25 minutes**

Answer to question one:
What is presbycusis and how will it affect Agnes' hearing?

Presbycusis is derived from two Greek words – presbus = old man and acusis = hearing. (see Useful Website)

Presbycusis is a sensorineural deafness that occurs with the normal ageing process. With presbycusis most people can hear speech but have difficulty in understanding it as speech as distortions occur (Mosby, 1994) because some of the high-pitched sounds (e.g. s, st, f, ph, ch) are filtered from normal speech. Hearing can also be reduced by accumulation of cerumen in the external auditory meatus.

Answer to question two:
Identify three other causes of sensorineural deafness.

- Noise-induced causes
- Menière's disease
- Ototoxic drugs
- Labyrinthitis
- Congential syphilis
- Hereditary disease
- Acoustic neuralgia
- Maternal rubella.

Answer to question three:
Name the other type of hearing loss and identify three causes.

Conductive deafness

- Wax
- Trauma
- Congenital causes
- Otitis media
- Otosclerosis
- Eustachian tube obstruction.

Answer to question four:
Explain the care of a hearing aid.

Cleaning – the connection hook and mould can be removed for cleaning by gently pulling them from the case. These can then be cleaned using warm, soapy water. Ensure that it is dry before using. The Cherry Rodenhever profile (p. 61) discusses the care of hearing aids.

If the hearing aid whistles, when in Agnes' ear, the noise is due to sound escaping from the ear, producing feedback. The ear mould is either poorly fitted or loose and should be adjusted.

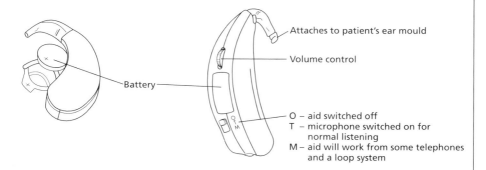

Attaches to patient's ear mould

Volume control

Battery

O – aid switched off
T – microphone switched on for normal listening
M – aid will work from some telephones and a loop system

Figure 22.1: Diagram of postaural hearing aid.

Answer to question five:
How could Agnes' ability to hear and understand what is communicated to her be improved?

Background noise such as cleaning work and loud television should be reduced. Ensure that you speak to Agnes so that *your face* is on the same level as hers, with the light on *your face* and look at Agnes when you are talking to her. This allows her the opportunity to lip read. Speak slightly more slowly and distinctively; do not cover your mouth and do not shout. Use the written word if necessary.

Use the 'T' position on Agnes' hearing aid if she is using the telephone. When visiting the theatre she should set the hearing aid to the 'T' position as many theatres and cinemas have induction loops that generate an electromagnetic field, which is received by the hearing aid and improves the quality of sound heard (Mosby, 1994).

Reference

Mosby's Medical, Nursing and Allied Health Dictionary (1994). (4th ed.) St Louis, MO: Mosby Year Book.

Further reading

Bond, M., Arthur, A., Avis, M. (1995). Distant voices. Nursing Times July 19: 91(29): 38–40.
Hines, J. (1997). Make the right noises caring for hearing-impaired patients. Nursing Times January 1: 93(1): 31–33.
Rye, S. (1990). A confusion of sound. Nursing Times September 12: 86(37): 43–44.

Useful Website

http://www.ukonline.co.uk/hearing.concern/fpres.htm (Accessed 2000, January 5)

Homosexuality: ageing process

Chris Buswell

Raymond and Henry have been a couple for 15 years. For the last 12 years they have lived together in Raymond's four-bedroomed detached house on the outskirts of town. Raymond is a 75-year-old bachelor, who formerly worked as a solicitor in a busy office in London. Henry, a retired accountant, is 68 years old and is a divorcee. Henry divorceed his wife 18 years ago. 'After the children grew up and left home,' he tells people. Henry had always thought himself to be bisexual, and by marrying had tried to deny his true sexuality to himself and others. However he began having a string of affairs, with men and women, 'About 10 years into a doomed marriage,' he reports.

Henry has no further contact with his wife. Since he moved in with Raymond, his two children have also ceased visiting their father. Raymond has no living relatives.

Due to advancing Parkinson's disease, Raymond finds climbing the stairs of their house difficult. Last year they decided to convert their downstairs study into a bedroom. Henry was pleased to have their bedroom downstairs as he also found climbing the stairs difficult. Chronic obstructive airways disease (COAD) had made him increasingly breathless as he climbed to the top of the stairs. Conveniently, there is a toilet next to the study, so Henry uses this at night since he often has to pass urine 3–4 times.

At the same time as moving their bedroom downstairs, Raymond and Henry decided to employ a home help to assist them to clean the house and cook their meals. Sadly, the first two home helps left their employment within weeks, because they were offended by the fact that Raymond and Henry share a bed.

Raymond decided to sell his stocks and shares that he had built up over the years and use the money to employ a full-time day carer and a night carer. He felt that these carers would be more professional and accept their sexuality. He also knew that Henry and he were in declining health and would need personal care as well as help with cooking meals and cleaning.

This situation worked well for a year or two but due to the rising costs of employing a carer from a reputable agency, and not having the full use of their house due to failing health, Raymond and Henry have decided to look into moving to a nursing home. They still wish to be together, in the same bedroom, although they now sleep in separate beds. Because of Henry's worsening COAD, he often becomes breathless, particularly at night, and needs to sleep sitting up. He also takes salbutamol nebulisers 6 hourly.

Despite not being entitled to income support and funding their own placement for a nursing home, Raymond and Henry have asked a social worker to help them find a suitable home where they can live together. The social worker readily agreed to help since Raymond and Henry have no family to help them search for a suitable home.

Question one: Outline changes in elderly men that may affect their sexual activity.

30 minutes

Question two: Describe homosexuality in the elderly.

30 minutes

Time allowance: **1 hour**

Answer to question one:
Outline the problems that Alison is experiencing due to her thyroxine deficiency, giving a rationale for them.

Tiredness and lethargy

Alison has been feeling tired and lacking in energy as she is deficient in thyroxine (T4) and triiodothyronine (T3) hormones secreted by the thyroid gland. Thyroxine is formed by the molecular addition of iodine to the amino acid tyrosine. T3 and T4 are required in the body to stimulate the consumption of oxygen and thus the metabolism of all cells and tissues in the body. Metabolic activity has therefore been reduced in Alison's case (Jordan & White, 1998). She has developed auto-antibodies, which have damaged functional thyroid tissue, and therefore secretion of the hormone from the gland has been deficient.

Goitre

The secretion of T3 and T4 is regulated by the release of thyroid-stimulating hormone (TSH) from the anterior pituitary gland. A negative feedback system operates in the body to control T3 and T4 secretion. If serum levels of thyroxine rise, this is detected in the hypothalamus and the pituitary is signalled to release less TSH.

Owing to the deficiency of T3 and T4 in the body, the pituitary gland has been secreting excessive TSH to stimulate increased secretion of thyroxine by the thyroid gland. As the functional thyroid tissue has been destroyed, the gland cannot secrete enough and responds to the excess TSH with hypertrophy (enlargement). This is visible as a swelling in the neck known as goitre (Franklyn, 1993).

Dry skin and vocal changes (hoarse voice)

Thyroxine helps to maintain sebaceous secretions in the skin, and a lack of it leads to dry skin as in Alison's case. The goitre restricts and compresses the movement of the vocal cords and can lead to difficulties in speech.

Weight gain and poor appetite

As Alison's metabolic rate has been reduced, fat has not been catabolised for energy requirements in the body. Anabolism proceeds at a reduced rate with thyroxine deficiency but faster than catabolism, and therefore she has been prone to weight gain (Jordan & White, 1998). Her body's requirements for energy have been less and this together with tiredness has reduced her appetite. Alison is likely to have had a slight increase in body weight with the birth of her first child, and it may take some time to get back to her previous normal weight. Breastfeeding her baby will assist her weight loss.

Cold intolerance

Thyroxine is required to increase metabolic rate to raise body temperature. With deficiency the body cannot adapt quickly enough to cold temperatures. Alison would find cold conditions uncomfortable very quickly (Franklyn, 1993).

Irregular menstrual cycle

Disrupted metabolic processes with a lack of thyroxine can lead to an irregular menstrual cycle. This may not be noticeable in Alison's case as breastfeeding will delay the onset of regular menstruation (Franklyn, 1993).

Constipation

Lower metabolic rate and poor appetite can lead to reduced peristalsis, leaving Alison prone to constipation.

Anaemia

Reduced metabolism, and poor appetite and intake of nutrients can lead to reduced erythropoesis. Alison is therefore likely to have developed a mild anaemia; this will have aggravated her tiredness.

Difficulty with childcare and breastfeeding

Alison may have experienced some difficulties with breastfeeding as her body's overall milk production may have been reduced by the thyroxine deficiency. This is more often attributable to poor appetite and metabolism rather than milk production, which is, stimulated by female sex hormones, mainly prolactin (Diehl, 1998). Alison's tiredness is however likely to have been exacerbated by meeting the needs of her new baby.

Low self-esteem

Alison is very likely to have experienced this. Her perception may have been that she was always tired and found it difficult to cope with her new baby's demands. She may have seen other mothers who were less tired and felt she was not coping well.

Answer to question two:

How should Alison be advised about her condition and its future management, considering her initial misdiagnosis, and what information should be given to her?

Alison is likely to feel somewhat aggrieved by the late diagnosis of her condition and will possibly have lost some confidence in the primary health care team. Careful explanation of her condition is therefore essential.

Initially the nurse should ensure Alison understands the nature of her condition and its treatment with oral thyroxine replacement therapy. It should be explained that it commonly affects women more than men (particularly after childbirth) and that as antithyroid antibodies have damaged her thyroid gland, she will always need to take thyroxine (T4) tablets.

The nurse should reassure Alison that her care of her child has been in no way substandard, and that the levels of tiredness she is experiencing are due to her deficiency of T4 and will improve with replacement therapy. She should be told the condition does not affect her baby and that thyroxine levels will not be passed on in breast milk (Thyroid Foundation of America, 1999).

It should be emphasised that her level of tiredness should not in any way be equated with her ability to look after her baby and that she should soon start to feel better. It may well come as some relief to Alison that although she can be expected to be tired with a new baby, she should not feel as ill as she has been.

Alison is likely to be apprehensive about her changed physical appearance. She should be reassured that her weight should begin to reduce (although some change following childbirth may be apparent) and that her throat swelling and dry skin should return to normal once replacement therapy is established. She should be told that this may take several months (Franklin, 1993).

Alison should be encouraged to eat a balanced diet, paying particular attention to protein, vitamins and calcium whilst she is breastfeeding. She should be encouraged to discuss her diet with the health visitor if she has any queries.

The dose and nature of her replacement therapy should be discussed in detail. It should be emphasised that she will need periodic blood tests to check her T4 levels, especially initially to establish the ideal dosage.

The importance of ensuring that she does not run out of the drug should be emphasised as she must avoid omitting doses; for this reason, care will need to be taken when she is travelling to ensure she has a sufficient supply.

Alison should be encouraged to ask any questions she may have about her condition and given details of contacts, and patient information leaflets to help explain it.

She may ask if alternatives to daily tablets are available, such as monthly injections. She should be informed that this is not possible at present.

Alison is likely to ask if it will affect her driving licence or insurance. Although it does not affect her driving licence, it should be suggested that Alison contact her insurers and any other companies with which she has personal insurance. She should investigate if she needs to inform them of her changed health status. This will ensure she does not invalidate any policies she has by failing to disclose changes.

References

Diehl, K. (1998). Thyroid dysfunction in pregnancy. Journal of Perinatal and Neonatal Nursing 11(4): 1–12.

Franklyn, J. (1993). Hypothyroidism. Medicine International 21(5): 161.

Goldsmith, C. (1997). Hypothyroidism: easy to treat but often overlooked. NurseWeek California 10(22): 12–13.

Jordan, S., White, J. (1998). Systems and diseases. The endocrine system; hypothyroidism. Nursing Times 94(29): 50–53.

The Thyroid Foundation of America, Inc. (1999). Thyroid disease after childbirth. http://www.clark.net/pub/tfa/brochure/brochure-post.html [Accessed 22/10/99].

Further reading

Walsh, M. (1997). Watson's Clinical Nursing & Related Sciences. (5th ed.). London: Baillière Tindall.

Taylor, C., Lillis, C., LeMone, P. (Eds) (1997). Fundamentals of Nursing: the Art and Science of Nursing Care. Cheltenham: Stanley Thornes Ltd. (Lippincott).

Useful Website

EndocrineWeb
http://endocrineweb.com
((1999) maintained by YourDoctor Inc.)

References

Bond, J., Coleman, P., Peace, S. (1993). Ageing in Society: An Introduction to Social Gerontology. (2nd ed.). London: Sage Publications Ltd.

Christiansen, J.L., Grzybowski, J.M. (1993). Biology of Aging. St Loius, Mosby-YearBook Inc.

Hocking, J. (1999). Continence problems: how to tackle reticence of patients. Nursing Times 95(1): 56–58.

Iqbal, P., Castledine, C.M. (1997). The management of urinary incontinence in the elderly. Gerontology 43(3): 151–157.

Mahony, C. (1997). The impact of continence problems on self-esteem. Nursing Times, 93 (52), 58–60.

Norton, C. (1996). (Ed.). Nursing for Continence. London: The Continence Foundation.

Resnick, N.M. (1993). Geriatric medicine and the elderly patient. In: Tierney, M. (Ed.). Current Medical Diagnosis and Treatment. Norwalk, Connecticut: Appleton & Lange.

Roper, N., Logan, W., Tierney, A. (1996). The Elements of Nursing. (4th ed.). Edinburgh: Churchhill Livingstone.

Torrance, C., Jordan, S. (1995). Bionursing: assessment of stress incontinence. Nursing Standard 10(4): 29–31.

Thayer, D. (1994). How to assess and control urinary incontinence. American Journal of Nursing October 1994: 42–47.

Further reading

Miller, C.A. (1995). Nursing Care of the Older Adult. Theory and Practice. (2nd ed.) Philadelphia: J.B. Lippincott Company.

Useful addresses

The Continence Foundation
307 Hatton Square
16 Baldwin Gardens
London EC1N 7RJ
Tel: 020 7404 6875

Association for Continence Advice
Winchester House
Kenning Park
Cranmer Road
London SW9 6EJ
Tel: 020 7820 8113

Infestation and pet residence in a rest home for elderly people

Tinuade Okubadejo

Susan Johnson, the manager of a rest home, has contacted the district nurse attached to the home because several residents have been complaining of an itchy, red 'rash' mainly on their ankles. It is May and, as the temperature has increased over the past few days, the problem has become worse. With medical involvement, the problem is diagnosed to be flea-bites from an adopted stray cat, named Felicity. Miss Cooke, who is 82 years old and quite frail, is one of the residents on the ground floor. She began feeding the cat several months ago, encouraging it into her room, and has taken it to the veterinary surgery once for various treatments.

The cat has subsequently become a favourite in the home. She is very placid, friendly and affectionate to the residents, who have commented that they feel much better since her arrival. She has made the home her territory and has taken to sleeping on the residents' beds, particularly that of Miss Cooke, who encourages the cat to do so. However, the flea outbreak has upset people very much. Miss Cooke feels very guilty about the incident, but is distraught by the thought of the cat being taken away. She has her venous leg ulcers dressed by the community nurse and declared this morning in great distress that if Felicity had to go, she could 'see no point in carrying on'. Miss Cooke, in addition to bites on her ankles, has bites on her trunk and arms.

Mrs Jones wants some advice as to what to do, because some of the residents' relatives think the cat should be put down, whilst the residents themselves are threatening to leave the home if the cat is removed from the premises! The nurse is aware from her visits that all the residents are unanimous in wishing to keep the cat; whilst the frailer and less mobile residents in particular, are benefiting from the presence of such an affectionate animal. At present, there is no one living or working in the rest home who has a chest condition or allergy to animals.

Question one: What are the health risks posed by this situation and how easily can it be controlled?

10 minutes

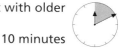

Question two: What are the benefits of animal involvement with older people?

10 minutes

Question three: What advice should the community nurse give in this case?

10 minutes

Time allowance: **30 minutes**

Answer to question one:
What are the health risks posed by this situation and how easily can it be controlled? (see Schmidt & Roberts, 1996).

Fleas, (the Siphonaptera family), are a type of parasite, living on blood. The species of pest involved in this case is *Ctenocephalides felis*, the cat flea, which prefers to live on a feline host; however, they will also attack other mammals, including humans if no cat is available. The foci of the outbreak are Felicity's sleeping places, because this is where the flea larvae are concentrated and develop.

Although irritating, flea bites are usually easily treated with a cooling lotion such as calamine or phenolated calamine; an antihistamine drug may be prescribed for a more severe reaction (Henry, 1994). Tea tree or lavender essential oils may also be used undiluted to relieve the rash (Lawless, 1992).

It will be necessary to treat any affected bedding that Felicity has been sleeping on; both pet and human bedding and clothing should also be checked, particularly the seams, for fleas. Both clothing and bedding may be treated easily by a hot wash and tumble drying in domestic machines (Henry, 1994; Schmidt & Roberts, 1996). Advice should be sought from a pest-control agency and the veterinary surgery that the cat attends, since treatment of carpets will be necessary.

If the residents wish to keep the cat, she should be fitted with a flea collar of slow-release vapours, treated with a long-acting spray or given oral medication to render any flea eggs infertile. She should also be provided with a special sleeping area so that any potential breeding sites are minimised. Additionally, it would be possible to use a 'flea-trap', a device emitting light that is fitted with a yellow-green filter, which attracts fleas (Schmidt & Roberts, 1996).

Answer to question two:
What are the benefits of animal involvement with older people?

Pet animals can have a truly beneficial effect on older people's psychological and physiological health overall, which may outweigh the risks of infections and the risk of bereavement should the animal die (Jarvis, 1997; Phillip, 1998). Petting and caring for an animal can induce a state of relaxation, a general feeling of well-being, and the reduction of loneliness, anxiety and depression (Dolan, 1997; Jarvis, 1997; Jennings, 1997; Willis, 1997), which lead to a much improved quality of life for older people.

Answer to question three:
What advice should the community nurse give in this case?

From a health point of view, Felicity could stay in the home with proper action taken to ensure that she remains free of fleas. For example, Miss Cooke might wish to take on the responsibility of grooming her with a close-toothed comb and it would be necessary to clean the carpets and seats in the home daily. This would mean residents would have to ensure that they keep floors clear to permit thorough cleaning.

There are benefits to some of the residents that could be very worthwhile. However, consideration also needs to be given to any residents or staff who dislike or are allergic to cats for any reason, particularly those with pre-existing respiratory conditions such as asthma or chronic obstructive airways disease.

Since in this instance, there are no reasons not to keep the cat, if this decision is taken, there are implications for marketing. The home should include in its publicity the fact that it accepts pets; the vast majority of residential homes in the UK do not do so (Jarvis, 1997; Phillip, 1998). This could become a selling point and a means of ensuring the home's financial survival, since there are many elderly people wishing to take pets with them to more suitable homes (Phillip, 1998). The Cinnamon Trust keeps a register of residential and nursing homes that accept pets along with their owners (Jarvis, 1997). The residential home could be added to this register. Potential employees and residents should be made aware of the home's status with respect to pets.

References

Dolan, M. (1997). Home Rx: wet nose, soft fur and wagging tail. Nursing October: 27(10): 12–13.
Henry, J. (Ed.). (1994). The British Medical Association New Guide to Medicines and Drugs. (3rd ed.). London: Dorling Kindersley.
Jarvis, A. (1997). Animal action stations. Nursing Times May 14: 93(20): 66.
Jennings, L.B. (1997). Potential benefits of pet ownership in health promotion. Journal of Holistic Nursing December: 15(4): 358–372.
Lawless, J. (1992). The Encyclopaedia of Essential Oils. Shaftesbury, Dorset: Element Books.
Phillip, J. (1998). Friends in need. The Guardian newspaper, May 6: p. 6.
Schmidt, G.D., Roberts, L.S. (1996). Foundations of Parasitology. (5th ed.). London: Wm C. Brown Publishers.
Willis, D.A. (1997). Animal therapy. Rehabilitation Nursing March–April: 22(2): 78–81.

Further reading

The Anchor Trust (1998). Losing a Friend To Find a Home.
Dossey, L. (1997). The healing power of pets. Alternative Therapies In Health and Medicine July: 3(4): 8–16.
Heath, S. (1999). Duty and the beasts. Nursing Times April 14: 95(15): 32–33.
Jarvis, A. (1997). Ageing matters. Nursing May 14–20: 93(20): 66.
Lowe, J. (2000). Are you up to scratch? Nursing Times Jan 20: 96(3): 51–52.
Robinson, I. (1999). Pet therapy. Nursing Times April 14: 95(15): 33–34.

Useful addresses

The Anchor Trust
Tel: 01865 854000

The Cinnamon Trust (Director: Averil Jarvis)
Foundry House
Foundry Square
Hayle
Cornwall TR27 4HH
Tel: 01736 757900
Fax: 01736 757010

Laryngectomy: communication, multidisciplinary team, body image

Barbara Marjoram

George Haven, a 63-year-old, lives with his wife Dorothy, who is 58, in their three-bedroomed house in the centre of town. He retired as a school teacher last year, taking the opportunity of early retirement. They have good neighbours and friends who are very supportive of them. Their three children, one daughter and two sons, have their own families, the nearest living 30 miles away. Their daughter visits them once a month and their sons try to visit two to three times a year.

George's hobbies include singing in the church choir and making miniature figures and buildings for train sets, something he started when his first grandchild was born 15 years ago. Dorothy works as a librarian in the local school and has no plans to retire for several years. She enjoys reading, furnishing her Victorian dolls' house and, when the weather is good, gardening.

George has smoked 10 cigarettes a day for many years and he enjoys a whisky as a nightcap. He has enjoyed good health all his life, only suffering from the usual childhood illnesses, e.g. chickenpox, measles and mumps, as well as an appendicectomy 50 years ago. However, over the last 6 months he complained of a persistent sore throat and hoarseness of voice, for which he visited his GP. The GP prescribed antibiotics that did not resolve the condition. He did not return to his GP until last week, after he developed earache. He was referred to the Ear, Nose and Throat (ENT) consultant for further investigations.

George's diagnosis has been confirmed as cancer of the larynx, involving his vocal cords and extending into the supraglottic region. George was then admitted for a laryngectomy.

George underwent surgery consisting of a total laryngectomy and thyroidectomy, with preservation of the parathyroid glands.

Question one: Why was George at risk of developing cancer of the larynx?

Question two: What invasive investigations should the ENT consultant undertake?

Question three: What are the differences between a tracheotomy, tracheostomy and laryngectomy?

Question four: What members of the multidisciplinary team should be involved in George's pre- and postoperative care?

Question five: The laryngectomy stoma forms an artificial airway that bypasses the physiological/protective functions of the nose, mouth and pharynx. How will this affect George and how can the physiological/ protective problems be overcome?

Question six: How often should endotracheal suction be performed on George and how often should the catheter be inserted?

Question seven: Prior to discharge, what knowledge and advice will George and his wife require?

Question eight: What changes will George, postlaryngectomy, have to adapt to and how might these affect him and his lifestyle?

Question nine: a) How did George produce 'normal' speech, before surgery?

b) How will he communicate after the laryngectomy?

Time allowance: **30 minutes**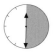

Answer to question one:
Why was George at risk of developing cancer of the larynx?

In the UK, cancer of the larynx in males represents approximately 1% of all malignancies; in females the percentage is lower (Harding, 1994). As Scott-Brown (1987 cited in Harding, 1994) identified, George would be more at risk because he smokes and drinks alcohol.

Answer to question two:
What invasive investigations should the ENT consultant undertake?

- Indirect laryngoscopy under local anaesthetic
- Direct laryngoscopy and biopsy under general anaesthetic.

Answer to question three:
What are the differences between a tracheotomy, tracheostomy and laryngectomy?

- *Tracheotomy* is an incision into the trachea through the neck below the larynx. It can be performed as an emergency or planned procedure. The tracheotomy is performed by making a small hole in the fibrous tissue of the trachea and a tracheostomy tube can then be inserted.
- *Tracheostomy* is an incision into the trachea through the neck and the larynx. It is performed by excising a small piece of the third tracheal ring, so fashioning the opening; a tracheostomy tube is then inserted. A tracheostomy is a planned procedure and can be temporary or permanent. Figure 27.1 is a diagram showing a tracheostomy.
- *Laryngectomy* is the surgical removal of the larynx and is performed to treat cancer of the larynx. The top of the remaining trachea is sutured to the skin, on the front of the neck, with a tracheal ring fashioning the opening. The remaining defects in the pharynx and oesophagus are sutured. (Mosby's Medical, Nursing and Allied Health Dictionary, 1994) Figure 27.2 shows a laryngectomy.

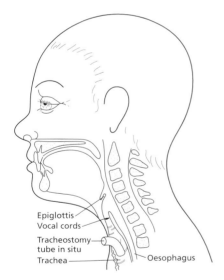

Figure 27.1: Diagram showing a tracheostomy.

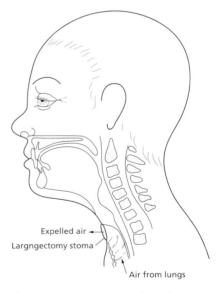

Figure 27.2: Diagram showing a laryngectomy.

Answer to question four:

What members of the multidisciplinary team should be involved in George's pre- and postoperative care?

- Nurse
- Physiotherapist
- Speech therapist
- Doctor
- Dietician
- District nurse.

Answer to question five:

The laryngectomy stoma forms an artificial airway that bypasses the physiological/protective functions of the nose, mouth and pharynx. How will this affect George and how can the physiological/protective problems be overcome?

The nose has a warming, humidifying and filtering effect on the air inspired.

The respiratory tract has a ciliated membrane, a local immune system and the cough reflex to protect the airway. These are necessary for the destruction of micro-organisms and the removal of debris from the lungs (Ashurst, 1992). However a laryngectomy bypasses these protective functions and inhibits the cough reflex. As Odell et al (1993) identified, if air is allowed to be inspired through the laryngectomy without first warming, humidifying and filtering it, the drying effect on the tracheobronchial mucous membrane causes the cilia to become paralysed. This causes a decrease in the effectiveness of the normal protective mechanisms of the respiratory tract and therefore George will become more vulnerable to opportunist infections. As Ackerman (1985 cited in McEleney, 1998) identified, there is an increase in mucous secretions and a reduction in pneumocytes and surfactant, which causes an effect on gaseous exchange and elasticity of the pulmonary tract. This mucous secretion is often thick and tenacious, so it will probably make it difficult for George to expectorate (Ashurst, 1992).

To overcome these problems George will require warmed, humidified air and tracheal suction until his respiratory tract adapts to the changes. Once he no longer requires mechanical humidification, George can wear a 'laryngectomy bib' around his neck. This can be dampened and therefore allows inspired air to be humidified and filtered.

Answer to question six:
How often should endotracheal suction be performed on George and how often should the catheter be inserted?

Tracheal suctioning should only be undertaken when clinical signs and symptoms dictate (Mancininelli-Van Atta & Beck, 1992) because of the risk of mucosal trauma, which can occur during suctioning.

Deppe et al (1993) identified that colonisation of the tracheobronchial tree with antibiotic-resistant Gram-negative flora is a risk factor for nosocomial pneumonia. As the normal protective mechanisms are bypassed in patients with tracheostomies and laryngectomies, there is a risk of infection. As Knox (1993) identified, there is a potential for introducing infective pathogens into the respiratory tract when suctioning is performed. It is therefore important that tracheal suction should be performed aseptically. To help reduce the risk of reintroducing micro-organisms into the respiratory tract during suctioning, a sterile catheter must be used for each insertion.

Answer to question seven:
Prior to discharge, what knowledge and advice will George and his wife require?

- Confirm that George and family can perform laryngectomy care
- Confirm that George and family can operate associated equipment
- Ensure George and family know contact numbers in case he/they require assistance
- Confirm that George has follow-up speech therapy appointments
- Confirm that George has follow-up outpatients appointments.

Answer to question eight:
What changes will George, postlaryngectomy, have to adapt to and how might these affect him and his lifestyle?

- Loss of voice
- Alteration to the 'normal' airway
- Disfigurement.

Minear and Lucente (1979 cited in Feber, 1996) and Byrne et al (1993) identify that a substantial number of patients postlaryngectomy experience poor psychological adjustment and depression following the surgery. Price (1990) suggests that body image consists of three central components – body reality, body ideal and body present. Body image, he suggests, is a mental picture which is dynamic and is adjusted regularly both in health, injury and illness. Devins et al (1994) suggested that patients postlaryngectomy, because of their 'unusual' voice, felt stigmatised in social situations and this had a negative impact on their quality of life.

George may experience grief, denial and anger, which are all part of the grieving process (Kubler-Ross, 1969). George may deny the laryngectomy or project anger on to those around him as he adjusts to his new body image.

George has lost the ability to communicate effectively as the loss of voice and the ability to speak is very debilitating. Ulbricht (1986 cited in Feber, 1996) identifies that with a laryngectomy, George will not be able to make the sounds of shouting, crying or laughing. Jay et al (1991) noted that 45% of patients felt that they were less socially acceptable after laryngectomy surgery. George may fear rejection by his family and friends because of the excretion (mucous) that is expectorated from the stoma.

Answer to question nine:

a) How did George produce 'normal' speech, before surgery?

b) How will he communicate after the laryngectomy?

a) During speech the vocal cords tighten and move closer together. Air from the lungs is then forced between them so that they vibrate, therefore producing sound. The lips, teeth and tongue all help to form the words.

b) He will communicate after the laryngectomy by one of the following methods:

1. Oesophageal speech
2. Electronic device (electrolarynx)
3. Transoesophageal valve.

Stam et al (1991) noted that males are more likely to learn oesophageal speech than females because they find the deep throaty voice less embarrassing. Postlaryngectomy, George will be inhaling and exhaling air via a permanent stoma site in his neck. In oesophageal speech air is swallowed and allowed to escape via 'burping' in a controlled fashion. This air escape causes the walls of the oesophagus to vibrate, which produces sound and is then articulated by the mouth and lips to produce speech (see Useful Websites).

The electronic device is hand held and is approximately the size of a small shaver. It has a vibrating plastic diaphragm so that George can use it to

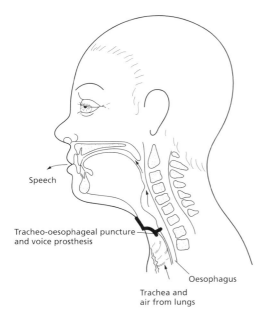

Speech

Tracheo-oesophageal puncture and voice prosthesis

Oesophagus

Trachea and air from lungs

Figure 27.3: Tracheo-oesophageal voice prosthesis.

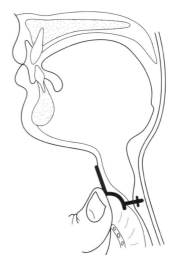

Figure 27.4: Stoma closed with thumb: low pressure prosthesis shown.

communicate by holding the electronic device against his neck, turning it on and articulating with his tongue, palate, throat and lips. This causes the diaphragm to vibrate, which produces a vibration in his throat that duplicates the vibration of the vocal chords. This device produces a very mechanical tone that has an unnatural sound to it (see Useful Websites).

For George to be able to communicate using the transoesophageal valve method, a small opening (fistula) is created between the trachea and oesophagus. A small valve is placed into the opening; this is a small tube with a non-return valve so that air can be directed into the oesophagus, but no air, food or fluid can enter the trachea. Figure 27.3 shows the positioning of a tracheoesophageal voice prosthesis. In order for George to talk, he will need to cover the stoma with his thumb during expiration, forcing air from the trachea into the oesophagus. Figure 27.4 shows how the stoma is closed with the thumb. A low-pressure prosthesis is shown. This produces sound, which is then enhanced by the lips and tongue through 'normal' articulation, so producing near-normal speech (see Useful Websites).

References

Ackerman, M.H. (1985). The use of bolus normal saline installations in artificial airways: is it useful or necessary? Heart and Lung 14: 505–506. In: McEleney, M. (1998). Endotracheal suction. Professional Nurse March: 13(6): 373–376.

Ashurst, S. (1992). Suction therapy in the critically ill patient. British Journal of Nursing 1(10): 485.

Byrne, A. Walsh, M., Farrelly, M., O'Driscoll, K. (1993). Depression following laryngectomy. British Journal of Psychiatry August: 163: 173–176.

Deppe, S.A., Kelly, J.W., Thoi, L.L. et al. (1993). Incidence of colinization, nosocomial pneumonia and mortality in critically ill patients using Trach closure system versus an open suction system: prospective randomised study. Critical Care Medicine 18(12): 1389–1393.

Devins, G.M., Stam, H.J., Koopmans, J.P. (1994). Psychosocial impact of laryngectomy mediated by perceived stigma and illness intrusiveness. Canadian Journal of Psychiatry 39(10): 608–616.

Harding, E. (1994). Preparing patients for the effects of laryngectomy. Nursing Times August 10: 90(32): 36–37.

Jay, S., Ruddy, J., Cullen, R.J. (1991). Laryngectomy: the patient's view. Journal of Laryngology and Otology 105(11): 934–938.

Knox, A.M. (1993). Performing endotracheal suction on children: a literature review and implications for nursing practice. Intensive and Critical Care Nursing 9(1): 48–54.

Kubler-Ross, E. (1969). On Death and Dying. London: Tavistock/Routledge.

Mancininelli-Van Atta, J., Beck, S.L. (1992). Preventing hypoxemia: haemodynamic compromise related to endotracheal suctioning. American Journal of Critical Care 1(3): 62–79.

Minear, D., Lucente, M.D. (1979). Current attitudes of laryngectomy patients. Laryngoscope 89: 1061–1065. In: Feber, T. (1996). Promoting self-esteem after laryngectomy. Nursing Times July 24: 92(30): 37–39.

Mosby's Medical, Nursing and Allied Health Dictionary (1994). (4th ed.). St Louis, MO: Mosby Yearbook.

Odell, A., Allder, A., Bayne, R. et al. (1993). Endotracheal suction for adult non-head-injured patients: a review of the literature. Intensive and Critical Care Nursing 9(4): 274–278.

Price, B. (1990). A model for body image care. Journal of Advanced Nursing 15(5): 585–593.

Scott-Brown, W.G. (1987). Otolaryngology. London: Butterworth. In: Harding, E. (1994). Preparing patients for the effects of laryngectomy. Nursing Times August 10: 90(32): 36–37.

Answer to question two:
What is the method of treatment and value of larval therapy for Miss Flanagan?

Larval therapy, using sterile maggots from greenbottle flies, is not a new discovery. Military surgeons reported that infested wounds did not get infected; gangrene and tetanus were not apparent in these wounds either. Its use was reported as long ago as the American Civil War (Chernen, 1986).

How larval therapy works

Small, sterile maggots, about 1–2 mm in length, are put onto the wound. It has been recommended that no more than 10 maggots, per cm^2, should be used, as too many will cause irritation (Waters, 1998). The larva are placed on a sterile net; this permits oxygen to permeate through, but prevents the maggots from escaping. An absorbent dressing is then put over the area and is fastened with tape.

The maggots produce strong proteolytic enzymes, which cause the necrotic tissue to disintegrate into a semi-liquid state. It is used by the larvae as food and is sucked up into their gut to be digested with the bacteria from the wound. In this way, the necrotic tissue is removed, whilst further infection and unpleasant odours are kept at bay.

It has also been stated by Waters (1998) that larval therapy can reduce wound pain and stimulate the formation of granulation tissue. Frequent changes of dressing are necessary, as copious amounts of exudate are produced, which may cause the maggots to drown or suffocate.

The larvae are removed by flushing with water or the use of forceps after a maximum of 3 days in situ. The maggots will try to leave the wound site in order to pupate and will be very active. They migrate to the surface of the wound, from where they are easy to remove. New maggots, for reapplication, may be needed. The old larvae are sent to pathology for examination.

Figure 28.1 shows maggots used for larval therapy.

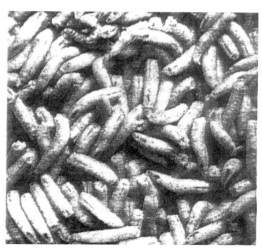

Figure 28.1 Use of maggots in larval therapy.

NB: The greenbottle fly *Lucilia sercata* is used to lay eggs on raw liver. The eggs are cleaned and sterilised to kill off surface bacteria and are then ready to be dispatched in sterile flasks. Within 12–24 hours the eggs hatch into maggots, which are stored, with sufficient oxygen, for further use.

(Jones & Champion, 1998)

Miss Flanagan understood the need for larval therapy, but like many patients, did not want to see what was going to be done or to see the larvae. Her only wish was for her leg ulcer to heal. Most people believe that the maggots will be identical in size and shape to fishing maggots, but in fact they are very small and once the results are seen, patients are usually converted to the benefits of their use.

Miss Flanagan did not experience pain or any sensation that the larvae were present. Three applications were needed before the ulcer was fully free of necrotic tissue. Conventional forms of treatment were then used, e.g. hydrogel and compression therapy.

In using larval therapy, Miss Flanagan would have had rapid wound debridement; unpleasant odours and pain would have been reduced. Larval therapy would also assist with the formation of granulation tissue (Thomas et al, 1996).

Answer to question three:
Once the venous ulcer is free from infection, what are the management priorities for Miss Flanagan's leg ulcer?

To focus entirely on the leg ulcer can be of little value. Miss Flanagan will need to give a detailed history of previous treatments, current drug therapy, allergies and risk factors for venous disease, such as previous limb trauma.

Miss Flanagan's social circumstances may also influence treatment outcomes; she lives alone, is female, and has a history of varicose veins, which all indicate that she is at high risk of further injury to her legs. Her nutritional state and ability to shop/cook will have to be assessed so that wound healing is not delayed by nutritional deficits, e.g. low levels of vitamin C.

The following questions should be asked and the answers dealt with:

- Is she compliant with her drug regimen?
- Is she comfortable with the use of larval therapy?
- Is larval therapy socially acceptable to her?
- Has she had enough education about this treatment and its effects?
- How does she regard the appearance of her leg in compression bandages?

The aim of treatment is to create an environment in which optimum healing can take place (Thomas, 1990).

The following tasks should be carried out:

Assessment

- Record measurements of size and shape of wound
- Record changes in state, i.e. colour (photographs can be used)
- Decide suitability of primary dressing (the appropriate dressing should be chosen for each stage of the healing process).

Treatment

- Bandages are irritants, so a layer of cotton, such as Tubifast, should be applied under the bandage, which will prevent direct contact with the skin
- A simple, effective emollient (50–50 cream, which consists of 50% white, soft paraffin and 50% liquid paraffin) is used to protect the skin from exudate
- Any eczema that may be present must be treated. Paste bandages, containing icthammol are useful on wet eczema
- Pain may be reduced by the use of compression bandages
- Elevation of the limb will also help to reduce pain
- Redness, heat and swelling may indicate the presence of cellulitis
- Systemic antibiotics may be used.

NB: The use of topical antibiotics can lead to multiresistant organisms and should therefore be avoided.

Education

- Miss Flanagan should be asked to take some form of regular exercise, give up smoking and lose weight, if necessary.
- Advice on how to elevate the leg when sitting should be given.
- The reasons for avoidance of standing for long periods, or sitting with the legs dependent, should also be given.
- Garters or tight socks should never be used as they will further restrict the circulation.
- Support stockings should be used once healing is complete.
- Regular checks on the healed limb are needed, at 6-monthly intervals.
- Protection against environmental hazards should be emphasised.

Social considerations

- It may be possible to get Miss Flanagan involved with her church, once again.
- When the pain and discomfort from her leg has gone, she may consider taking up teaching music, as before.
- Members of the local Women's Institute could be asked to call regularly.
- This may influence Miss Flanagan to restart attending regular monthly meetings. It may also lead to other social contacts, e.g. coffee mornings, outings etc.
- Regular contact with the local doctor's surgery is also needed.

References

Bosanquet, N. (1992). Cost of venous leg ulcers: from maintenance therapy to investment programmes. Phlebology 290 (Suppl 1): 44–46.

Cameron, J. (1995). Venous and arterial leg ulcers. Nursing Standard 9(26), 25–32.

Chernen, E. (1986). Surgical maggots. Southern Medical Journal 79(9): 1143–1145.

Jones, M., Champion, A. (1998). Nature's way. Nursing Times 94(34): 75–78.

Thomas, S. (1990). Wound Management & Dressings. London: The Pharmaceutical Press.

Thomas, S., Jones, M., Shutler, S. (1996). Using larvae in modern wound management. Journal of Wound Care 5(2): 60–69.

Waters, J. (1998). The benefits of larval therapy in wound care. Nursing Times 94(2): 62–64.

Losing a home

Vivienne Mathews

Lionel Peregrine-Jones, aged 85, lives in a large, isolated house in an upmarket suburb of London. He is a widower of 16 years' standing and is used to caring for himself. Lionel spent most of his life as a city stockbroker. He drove a Rolls Royce Silver Cloud; he went to Monte Carlo for his holidays and had a second home in Biarritz. He played golf and polo and gained an Olympic bronze medal for fencing in the 1934 Olympic games.

Pamela, his only daughter and a divorcee, has a prestigious job in London that involves commuting 80 miles a day and frequent trips abroad. Her only child, Martin, attends Keele University.

Lionel suffers from increasingly severe dementia, leading to a serious neglect problem of himself and his property. He is reluctant to accept help, allowing only Pamela and her son into the house at weekends. His anxiety stems from the fact that he has been burgled three times in quick succession and he is convinced that anyone entering the house is 'casing the joint' for future attacks.

Pamela visits on Saturdays when she can, doing a weekly shop to ensure frozen and tinned foods are available for her father. She is not at all sure what he eats.

The crisis point came when a small fire, caused by his drying his clothes too near the gas cooker, alerted neighbours to the danger Lionel was to them and to himself.

He is fiercely independent and does not want to leave his home and comfortable surroundings, but if persuaded by his daughter, may not resist being moved.

There are three choices open to Lionel and Pamela:

- For him to stay in his own home for as long as possible after activating all possible care services
- For him to go and live with his daughter
- For him to move into residential care.

Question one: What are the positive and negative benefits for Lionel and his daughter in:

1. Option one: staying in his own home
2. Option two: moving in with his daughter
3. Option three: moving into residential care

Time Allowance: **45 minutes**

Option one:
Staying in his own home

Mr Peregrine-Jones

This option would not involve any disruptive upheaval. He would continue to cope, after a fashion, in his own familiar surroundings, as he has always done. Importantly, his wishes would be respected.

As a result of his dementia, Lionel may be confused; he may find preparing meals a problem because of his poor sequencing abilities and short-term memory loss. Instructions will need to be written down in logical order. He will be unable to manage new skills, such as the use of a microwave oven, convenient and easy to use though it may be for him.

Lionel would continue to be anxious over his isolated state and repeated burglaries. He has become extremely vulnerable due to his increasing frailty. Visual and auditory problems will affect his ability to react when intruders or unwelcome callers are nearby. He would need to be encouraged to take appropriate measures to secure his living environment, e.g. remembering to lock doors, close windows and have a method of monitoring visitors (McMahon & Isaacs, 1997).

His only social contacts appear to be his neighbours, who would demonstrate a considerable degree of hostility towards him and so would not be supportive in any way. Lionel will be unable to understand and/or control his environment, which may lead to paranoid fears.

Pamela

She would not have to give up her independence by sharing her home with her father. She would, however, have to seek help on safety and security matters on her father's behalf. She could continue with her job with no constraints on time or movements. She may feel guilt, but could continue to be supportive with perhaps increased input into her father's situation. There would be the increased strain of travelling and even more guilt as the situation deteriorates further. There may be repercussions from her son at some time in the future.

Extensive domiciliary services would need to be mobilised, with increased pressure from the neighbours to 'get something done' about her father.

There may be consequent bad publicity for Social Services if Lionel was injured or killed in a possible fire or accident of some sort, but he would be independent and his identity and wishes would have been preserved.

NB: Community Care Act 1990.
The intention of the act is to help people lead independent lives in their own homes. Elderly people should have at their disposal a satisfactory amount of assistance and a say in how their lives should be governed and supervised.

(Harding, 1994)

Option two:
Living with his daughter

Mr Peregrine-Jones

Lionel may be angry at the forced move. He may be disorientated and no longer in control of his life. He would lose his independence and self-care abilities very quickly. He would have to master a new lifestyle (living with an undergraduate is not easy!), make new friends and may not recognise his own known local amenities, e.g. pub, library or supermarket. There would be a certain amount of antagonism from Martin over shared space, loud music, different foods to eat etc. Both Pamela and Martin will be out of the house for long periods of time, so what would Lionel do?

When memory is unreliable, even in a familiar environment, a change of residence may become extremely confusing and frightening. Simple things, such as finding the bathroom, can become a major concern. It would be very distressing for Lionel.

He would, of course, be physically safe; he would have regular social contact, a better diet, warmth, no worries about burglars or his decaying property. There would be no conflict with the neighbours.

> **NB:** Learned helplessness is a condition that occurs when a person encounters experiences that they feel they cannot control. It is common in old age and stems from dependency on others, so that if control is lost over where he is to live, Lionel will not be motivated to have control over other areas of his life.
>
> (Taylor & Field, 1993)

Lionel may feel a lack of control over this major event in his life, and may, therefore, fail to manage other aspects of his new life in which success is possible. He may deteriorate both physically and mentally.

Pamela

Pamela would find her job very difficult to maintain; she may have to give it up altogether and suffer the consequent lack of earning power. Having her father in the house would mean that, for Pamela, there would be loss of privacy, loss of freedom to come and go, and social relationships may suffer. The potential for the situation to deteriorate as the dementia worsens, is very real, and if this were the case, would Pamela continue to cope? Help could be given in the form of daily domestic work, personal care for her father and other chores, such as shopping and ironing. This is costly, and social services may not be able to help.

Pamela would, on the other hand, have freedom from guilt and anxiety about her father. She would not have to spend her weekends travelling to and from his house (a matter of 56 miles each way) doing his shopping, cleaning, laundry, etc.

Social Services would welcome this option as it is a cheaper solution for them, in the short term, but they should be aware that the situation may break down so more support would eventually be needed.

Option three:
Moving into residential care

Mr Peregrine-Jones

Once again, he would feel anger that his wishes had been disregarded; he would feel out of control, disorientated and his self-care skills would rapidly deteriorate as his loss of memory became more and more apparent. There would be reduced family contact. Whether he would mix with the other residents and fit in with group living where he had not taken part in any decision-making processes are relevant. Routines would be laid down by other people, e.g. what time to go to bed, what time to eat, visiting times, if restricted, etc. He would experience a loss of independence, privacy, and control over his environment.

Lionel would be physically safe, warm, well fed, and mentally stimulated. There would be plenty of social interaction with staff and other residents. He would not be a 'burden' to his daughter and her son and there would be no conflict with the neighbours (Norman, 1987).

Pamela

She would feel guilty that she 'put him away' or 'didn't do enough for him', which may cause her son to lose patience with her attitudes and regrets. Pamela knew her father's likes and dislikes, she tolerated his little idiosyncrasies as no one else could, and she could also get angry with him if she chose to and now cannot. She can only visit him at mutually convenient times. She may feel an element of dissatisfaction with the home, fitting into their routines and becoming an intruder on someone else's territory. Pamela may even be asked to wait outside the room while the carers bath and dress her father. She may find it difficult to ask if she can help (Harding, 1994). Feelings of disempowerment, of unspoken frustration that she should be treated like a stranger, will make her feel useless and may in time prevent her from visiting as often as she would like.

Care workers may feel that they are under scrutiny and be embarrassed as they perform tasks in front of Pamela.

Open discussion, initiated by the staff of the home, will go some way to clear the air and allow Pamela to ask questions, get involved with her father's care and begin to feel accepted as part of the caring team (McMahon & Isaacs, 1997).

NB: Relatives groups can be a useful way for relatives to express their feelings about their own situations and that of their loved ones. These shared experiences can be a great help in dispelling guilt and grief.

(McMahon & Isaacs, 1997)

Pamela may need time to express her anxieties and doubts about the admission of her father to long-term care. She may feel angry with herself and ambivalent about the home. It would be ideal if the staff included Pamela in their care planning decisions, and if she were consulted about her father's personality, habits and history, she would then feel valued.

Pamela's life – her job and her home – will be unchanged. There would be less travelling, more time for her family and her own persuits, and no more anxieties about Lionel's safety. The neighbours would be happy that 'something had been done!'

Which option would you choose?

References

Harding, J. (1994). Community care. In: McMahon, C.A., Harding, J. (Eds) Knowledge To Care: A Handbook for Care Assistants. Oxford: Blackwell Science, pp 237–245.

McMahon, C.A., Isaacs, R. (1997). Care of the Older Person: A Handbook for Care Assistants. Oxford: Blackwell Science.

Norman, A. (1987). Aspects of Ageism. London: Centre for Policy on Ageing.

Taylor, S., Field, D. (1993). Sociology of Health and Health Care. Oxford: Blackwell Science.

Further reading

Age Concern (1995). Caring for Older People at Home: Staff Guidelines. London: Age Concern.

Bender, M. (1995). An Active Solution for Health. Elderly Care 7(4): 20.

Useful addresses

Counsel & Care
Twyman House
16 Bonny Street
London NW1 9PG

Abbeyfield Society
Abbeyfield House
53 Victoria Street
Saint Albans
Herts HL1 3UW

Age Concern
82 Russia Lane
London E2 9LU

Manual handling: drag lift

Vivienne Mathews

'My dad is a big man; he weighs about 16 stone, I think. Mind you, that was before he "went off his legs," if you know what I mean! I expect he weighs more, now.

'He's in a nursing home and has a nice room with a lovely view of the docks, so's he can watch the ships come and go. It's the best I can do for him. I can't have him to live with me, not with four kids, two dogs, two rabbits and an unemployed husband! We haven't got the room and the khazi's upstairs anyway, so he couldn't manage to use that.

'"Harpo", as his friends used to call him, was in the navy for 28 years. He was the strong, silent type apparently. That's how he got his nickname, after Harpo Marx, you know, the silent one.

'My mum left him, and us, when he was invalided out of the navy. Couldn't put up with his malingering, I suppose. He used to say that his legs wouldn't work. Nor would he! Lived off his pension, some odd jobs and his betting.

'Now, of course, it's caught up with him. He can't walk, or stand, or bear his own weight for long. He has a wheelchair, but he doesn't like it as it's too small for him. He has great difficulty in moving up the bed or changing his position when he's slumped down in a chair.

'In the home, two nurses, big ones, take him by the armpits and heave him up the bed or chair. He shouts and yells that they are hurting him, but I don't see any other way of moving him. He's such a lump.

'He told me, the other day, that his bum was sore and that he thought there was some blood on the sheets after the last time the nurses moved him. Is that right? Can you help?'

Question one: What lift is Pearl describing? Describe the relevant legislation regarding manual handling of patients as they apply to Mr Harper.

15 minutes

Question two: In the manoeuvre described by Pearl, what are the risks to the patient and carers?

15 minutes

Question three: Suggest alternative ways that Mr Harper could be moved up the bed or chair.
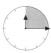
15 minutes

Time allowance: **45 minutes**

Answer to question one:
What lift is Pearl describing? Describe the relevant legislation regarding manual handling of patients as they apply to Mr Harper.

The lift being used on Clarence is a condemned lift known primarily as the 'drag lift' (Fig. 30.1). It is also called the 'underarm lift', the 'axilla lift', the 'auxiliary', the 'through arm lift' and, even, an 'assist'.

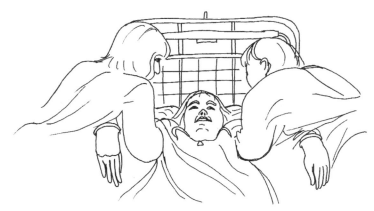

Figure 30.1: Drag lift.

The drag lift is any lift that involves moving the patient with the nurse's arms or hands under the patient's axilla. It can be done by one nurse (Fig. 30.2), producing a lopsided drag lift, but is more usually performed by two nurses working from the front. The drag lift has been outlawed since 1981, but can still be seen in hospitals, nursing homes, residential homes and in the community (Richmond, 1998).

According to Richmond (1998) it has proved to be a popular lift as the axilla acts as a 'natural handle' when moving a person.

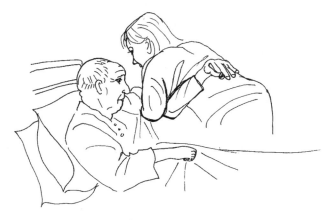

Figure 30.2: One-sided drag lift.

Legal requirements

There are five pieces of legislation relating to load management. These are:

1. Manual Handling Operations Regulations, 1992 . (MHO Regs).
2. The Management of Health and Safety at Work Regulations, 1992.
3. Regulations 5 to 7 of the Workplace (Health, Safety and Welfare) Regulations, 1992.
4. Health and Safety at Work Act (HASAWA), 1974.
5. The Reporting of Injuries, Diseases and Dangerous Occurrences Regulations, 1995. (RIDDOR) (Richmond, 1998).

Employers responsibilities

Under the Health and Safety at Work Act 1974, Reg 2, employers are responsible for the health, welfare and safety of their employees, and must provide instruction, supervision and training for them.

MHO regulations

Regulation 4 places responsibility on the employer in the following areas:

- Avoidance of manual handling
- Assessment of risks with reference to the following four main elements: (1) task; (2) load, (3) individual capacity, (4) working environment
- The reduction of risks with reference to the same four elements
- Provision of information on the load
- Review of risk assessment.

Regulation 5, of the Workplace (Health, Safety and Welfare) Regulations, 1992, deals specifically with the maintenance of the workplace and of equipment, devices and systems, placing responsibility on the employer to ensure that such are in efficient working order and in good repair.

Regulations 6–9 deal with the provision of adequate and appropriate ventilation, temperature, lighting and cleanliness.

Regulation 10 relates to room dimensions, giving minimum space allowances in which people are required to work (Richmond, 1998).

Employees' responsibility

Under the Health and Safety at Work Act, 1974, section 7, the employee is responsible for his own health, safety and welfare, and should cooperate with the employer to enable him to comply with health and safety duties.

Under the MHO Regulations, Regulation 5, the main responsibility of the employee is to make use of safe systems at work, provided by the employer.

Under the Management of Health and Safety at Work Regulations, 1992, Regulation 12, the responsibility of the employee is to use the equipment/

machinery/aids provided, in accordance with training and instruction given to the employee (Richmond, 1998).

All care workers should have a manual handling certificate stating that they are proficient in handling patients. This certificate should be updated annually. Mr Harper is being moved using a condemned lift, which must be changed immediately with appropriate handling equipment installed at the earliest opportunity.

Answer to question two:
In the manoeuvre described by Pearl, what are the risks to patients and carers?

Risk to patient

According to Holmes (1998):

- The drag lift is uncomfortable and dangerous to patients
- It hurts the patient because:
  - All the lifting force is applied to the soft tissues under the axilla
  - The force of this lift traps the soft tissue against the bone and causes pain and tissue damage
  - The brachial plexus, under the patient's arms, can be damaged
  - The shoulders can be dislocated
  - It contributes to the formation of pressure sores

NB: Tender skin can be damaged by friction and shearing forces, so that when the patient is left to lie on this area, a pressure sore will develop.

  - The patient can be dropped or injured

NB: All the patient's weight is on the nurses during this lift; if they lose control the patient and/or the nurse may well end up on the floor. It is all too easy to sustain injuries in this way.

  - It discourages the patient from mobilising (Holmes, 1998)

Risk to carers

The drag lift has six main faults (Holmes, 1998):

- The lift creates shearing forces across the shoulders
- The load (the patient) is taken at a distance from the base of the spine
- The lift involves a twist
- The patient tends to depend upon the carers for all support
- The carers have difficulty lowering a patient who collapses
- Often there is not enough space between wheelchair and chair, for example, to carry out this lift and carers may stumble

Answer to question three:
Suggest alternative ways that Mr Harper could be moved up the bed or chair.

First of all ask:

- Is the patient in the right type of bed/chair?
- Is the patient on the right type of mattress/cushion?
- Are there handling devices to complete the handling task?
- What techniques should be used?
- Is the environment safe for the handling task to be performed?

Secondly, once Mr Harper is sitting he should not be left unattended until he is comfortable and secure in the back of the chair seat.

Moving Mr Harper back in a chair

- If Mr Harper can use his arms he may be able to roll, or rock, from side to side, moving one buttock at a time back into the chair seat
- If there is a problem with weightbearing, a chair seat that slopes backwards, slightly, or a wedge under the seat cushion can be used
- When Mr Harper slumped forward in the chair, he could be encouraged to lean forward to the 'nose over toes' position; then use a rocking motion to push himself backwards into the seat (Holmes, 1998)
- Make sure there is enough room to move around the chair
- A handling belt could be useful in this situation; so could the use of a sliding board if transferring the patient from one chair to another or onto the bed from a chair
- A standing hoist is ideal for a non-weightbearing patient, but plenty of space is needed for this manoeuvre
- An armchair with a moveable arm may help with other handling techniques

> **NB:** Bobath technique
> Unless training in this technique has been undertaken, this type of procedure should not be used. Damage to patients and their carers can occur.

Moving a patient up the bed: equipment to use

- A hoist will reduce physical effort and strain on the carer
- A trapeze will not help the patient move up the bed; it is used for lifting and inserting a bedpan, for example, underneath the patient
- Patient-handling blocks allow a patient to help themselves by taking their own weight on their arms and so moving their buttocks up the bed
- A rope ladder allows the patient to pull themselves into a sitting position

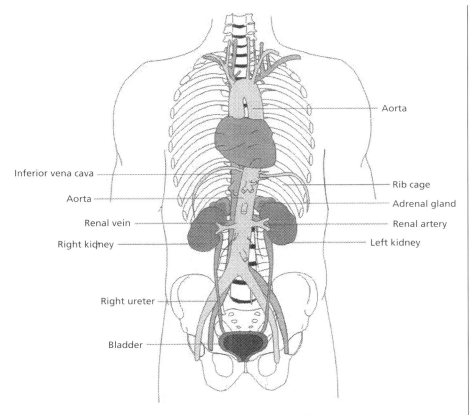

Figure 31.1: The kidneys and renal vessels within the body.

Answer to question one:
What possible developments in David's case could produce a life-threatening condition if the kidney was not removed?

Advanced necrosis of the kidney, or other internal structure, may produce toxins, which in turn could cause generalised septicaemia, septic shock and death (Hands & Morris, 1994).

Necrosis developing from the renal pelvis into the renal vessels may weaken them, permitting rupture and internal haemorrhage. Damage to the aorta or inferior vena cava is possible, with catastrophic results.

Persistent hypertension could give rise to a cerebrovascular accident or other major circulatory haemorrhage. The damaged kidney is likely to continue to produce renin in increased quantities, having a profound vasopressor effect (Smith, 1997).

Answer to question two:
In view of his general good health, what matters might be raised in the pre-operative phase from a nursing perspective?

Assessment of his condition showed that David was fit for surgery. Antibiotic therapy will need to be given to combat both existing kidney and nosocomial infections.

Care is needed with postoperative pain management, as pain is common following this procedure (Segal, 1996), and planning of breathing exercises, physical exercise and analgesics to limit pain should take place.

David should be warned that he may regain consciousness in a high-dependency unit (HDU), a common practice because of the major nature of the surgery, in order to monitor the initial recovery more closely, before returning to the ward. If time permits he might visit the HDU to increase his familiarity with it.

He should be advised that he will have venous access with i.v. fluids, and i.v. analgesia in situ when he wakens, as well as a urinary catheter and oxygen mask. He may be allowed to experience use of the mask prior to surgery to reduce his level of anxiety in using it.

He should be made aware that he might have breathing difficulty or discomfort following surgery, partly due to the proximity of the kidney to the diaphragm, and to possible pleural disturbance and removal of the 12th rib (often required in this procedure). To help him deal with this, ideally he should be instructed in, and allowed time to practice deep breathing exercises that will help his recovery. There may also be short-term spinal or pelvic discomfort due to his positioning on the table.

Answer to question three:
What are the initial priorities for this patient on returning to the ward?

Frequent observations of temperature, pulse, blood pressure and respiration rate will be required initially to note any tendency towards hypovolaemic shock, which could be sudden and catastrophic if any of the ligatures on the major vessels failed. The dressing should be checked for evidence of any excessive haemorrhage, and the drain should be checked to ensure that it is functioning correctly. The dressing and drain conditions must be recorded.

Temperature monitoring is necessary to detect any tendency to pyrexia, which might indicate the onset of infection, even though prophylactic antibiotics will be given routinely in theatre.

Radical nephrectomy is well known to be a painful procedure, and effective pain relief will require the use of IV narcotic analgesics initially (Segal, 1996). This is ideally administered using patient-controlled analgesia (PCA) once the patient has recovered sufficiently from the anaesthetic (Taylor et al, 1997). Effective pain control will reduce neuroendocrine stimulus, which causes raised blood pressure. This will further reduce the risk of postoperative haemorrhage and increase David's safety and comfort (Hands & Morris, 1994). The effectiveness of the pain relief should be monitored using a pain assessment tool, because prolonged or increasing pain could also indicate infection with delayed wound healing.

Observations of David's level of consciousness and respiratory rate are also necessary initially due to the respiratory depressive side-effects of narcotic analgesia. The respiration rate should not fall below about 8/minute. Potential respiratory problems arising from either the rib or pleural involvement in surgery must be observed for. David should be sat up as soon as possible, within the constraints of pain and its control, to assist breathing and the full expansion of the lungs. He should be encouraged to commence deep breathing exercises hourly, especially if he has been taught these pre-operatively.

Postsurgical physiotherapy will be arranged to help him drain and expectorate secretions. General mobilisation by physiotherapists and nurses should commence as early as possible.

Urinary catheter output and quality should be monitored to ensure David's remaining kidney is functioning well, there is no blood in the urine, which might suggest ligature leakage, and there is no infection. Wound drainage output should also be monitored to confirm satisfactory healing is taking place and to allow its earliest removal.

Peripheral hydration must continue until David is able to take oral fluids, and diet may recommence when bowel sounds are detected, indicating that peristalsis has returned.

Suggested further exercises

1. Investigate the current status of co-trimoxazole, and any alternatives in current use, using the British National Formulary, drug catalogues, or other appropriate materials.
2. Study pre-operative procedures where you work, anaesthetic fasting arguments, stress management techniques, and general pre-operative preparation.
3. Consider appropriate nutrition requirements in terms of tissue recovery, using texts on nutrition and wound care.

References

British National Formulary (current edition). London: British Pharmaceutical Press.

Droste, C., Von Planta, M. (1997). Clinical Medicine Memorix. London: Chapman & Hall.

Hands, L.J., Morris, P.J. (1994). In: Morris, P.J. (Ed.) The Oxford Textbook of Surgery. CD-ROM edition, Oxford: Oxford University Press.

Kerbl, K. (1993). Minimally invasive surgery – laparoscopic nephrectomy. British Medical Journal 307: 1488–1489.

McKinney, B. (1998). Hospital nursing – softening the edge of radical nephrectomy. Nursing 28(7): 32–34.

Marieb, E. (1998). Human Anatomy and Physiology. Harlow: Addison, Wesley, Longman.

Mawdsley, D. (1998). Urological Surgery. In: Simpson, P. (Ed.) Introduction to Surgical Nursing. London: Edward Arnold: pp 219–241.

Segal, S. (1996). Nursing rounds; radical nephrectomy (post-operative pain). American Journal of Nursing 96(7): 37–38.

Smith, T. (1997). Renal Nursing. London: Baillière Tindall.

Taylor, C., Lillis, C., LeMone, P. (1997). Fundamentals of Nursing: The Art and Science of Nursing Care. (3rd ed.). Lippincott, Cheltenham: Stanley Thomas Limited: p 1133.

Further reading

Rowett, H.G.Q. (1994). Basic Anatomy and Physiology. (3rd ed.). London: John Murray.

Nutritional assessment

Penelope Simpson

Layla Kaufmann, a frail widow of German–Jewish origin, is 81 and lives with her single daughter, Miriam, aged 48 and a freelance classical musician. They live in a second floor two-bedroomed inner city flat, with no lift. It is within walking distance of a small parade of shops. The synagogue is 3 miles away. Their neighbours and friends pop in several times a week, and the pair like entertaining. They have few relatives left alive. They belong to the local library and occasionally go to the theatre. They have no pets.

Layla was a reasonably successful author, and her husband, who died 15 years ago, was an accountant. He was English and Orthodox Jewish. They met in Germany and married immediately after the Second World War, and came to live in this country. She is small-boned, thin and suffers from arthritis and rheumatism, which means she does not get out much. She enjoys reading and does the crossword puzzle in her daily paper but has given up writing as she finds it hard to be creative anymore. She listens to music and watches certain television programmes avidly, arranging her life around her favourites. She likes several glasses of sherry a day 'to relax her'.

Miriam plays the violin and travels all over the country to concerts and to teach at schools, and in people's homes. She drives a Volvo and has done an advanced driving course, as she drives 2000 miles per month. She is short and inclined to be overweight, and her blood pressure is moderately elevated. She finds it difficult to fit exercise into her busy life and smokes about 30 cigarettes a day, mostly in her car, as her mother does not approve. She is beginning to worry about her mother's ability to cope without more formal support for when Miriam is away.

Question one: Layla and Miriam are practising Orthodox Jews. What dietary laws will be applied?

5 minutes

Question two: What factors need to be considered in maintaining an adequate nutritional intake for these women?

10 minutes

Time allowance: **15 minutes**

Answer to question one:
Layla and Miriam are practising Orthodox Jews. What dietary laws will be applied?

Judaism holds that all life, including that of animals, is held in great respect, so precise and rigorous rules apply to ensure that the animal's death is, as far as possible, instantaneous and painless. No animal that has died from disease or natural causes may be eaten. It is also forbidden to eat meat which is damaged in any way during slaughter, so pre-stunning is not allowed. Animals are killed by a specially trained person with a very sharp blade drawn across the throat, severing the airway and the blood vessels. The blood is drained as quickly as possible, and the meat salted and washed to remove all remaining traces. The resulting meat is called kosher, which means ritually fit in Hebrew. Only the meat of animals with cloven hooves and that chew the cud may be eaten; for example, lamb, beef, venison, and goat. Meat from the pig is forbidden, as is the sciatic nerve or hindquarters of any animal, so ham, bacon and pork sausages would be ruled out.

Herbivorous birds, such as chicken, duck, turkey, goose, pheasant and their eggs are permitted, but eggs are discarded if the smallest speck of blood is noted on the yolk. They may not eat shellfish or any fish without fins or scales. A specified time (between 3 and 6 hours) must elapse between the eating of meat and dairy products. Only half an hour is needed between taking dairy products and then meat.

Separate storage, preparation and cooking areas, serving utensils and crockery are needed for meat and milk products, even down to the dishwasher. In effect, two separate kitchens are needed (Shamash, 1998). Kosher pure vegetable margarines and vegetable oils may be used when cooking meat. Food prepared by gentiles is not kosher and may not be acceptable. Kosher wines are available for ritual purposes, but there are no other restrictions on alcohol.

During Pesach (Passover), which is in March/April, all leavened foods, agents, and any utensils used to prepare them may not be used. Unleavened bread (Matzo) made from wheat and water is eaten instead. Devout Jews may fast for 25 hours at the feast of Yom Kippur, which takes place in September/October (Fieldhouse, 1995).

If they conform to dietary laws, they could be eating a reasonably balanced diet. Chicken soup, made the Jewish way, has been shown to boost the immune system.

Answer to question two:
What factors need to be considered in maintaining an adequate nutritional intake for these women?

Financial factors

Layla may have financial problems such as a limited old age pension available. Miriam may have a fairly hand-to-mouth existence as a freelance, possibly self-employed musician, so money may be tight for the pair of them.

Social factors

A frail 81-year-old may not have the abilities to shop and cook for herself if her daughter is away for any length of time. As an immigrant, she may not have family/friends/neighbours willing and able to help out. Her friends may have 'died off' and she may feel isolated and depressed. Her family may have been lost in the Holocaust.

Historical, political, cultural and psychological factors

Layla may have fixed or old fashioned notions of what she should eat. She may have longstanding mental or physical health problems arising from the two World Wars. She was born during the First World War (1914–1918), which Germany lost. Antisemitism was rife between these two wars and persecution was possible. She was in her early 20s when the Second World War started; she may have been interned, starved, tortured, worked almost to death or even experimented on (Shamash, 1998). As a result she was unlikely to have achieved maximum skeletal density.

Physical factors

Layla is at risk of osteoporosis, so it would be useful to check her calcium and vitamin D intake. She is at higher risk if she is small and thin, has lost weight recently, drinks a lot of alcohol and/or takes little weightbearing exercise due to fragility or depression (Simpson, 1999). She may not go out much, and as vitamin D is synthesised by the action of sunlight on skin, this could be a problem for her. To gain this benefit, 20 minutes/day of full-spectrum daylight is needed.

Miriam is at risk of heart disease or hypertension if her mother was malnourished during her pregnancy.

She is reaching the age when her teeth are becoming unreliable and she may not chew food properly. Her mother's dentures may not fit too well if her frailness means that she has lost weight. Neither women may have the money or time for proper dental care. Layla may find that her arthritis makes it difficult for her to chew food adequately. She may also notice that her ability to taste and smell food has diminished (Griep et al, 1996), lessening her enjoyment of it, and perhaps reducing her intake.

Miriam may find it hard to fit in a healthy balance of diet and exercise with her work, particularly when she travels, or with looking after her mother. Her basal metabolic rate (Webb & Copeman, 1996) has been slowing since her 20s, so she may be noticing an increasing tendency to put on weight.

The four essential questions to ask when screening for nutritional status are:

1. Have you unintentionally lost weight recently?
2. Have you been eating less than usual?
3. What is your normal weight?
4. How tall are you?

(Norton, 1996)

Their knowledge of a healthy diet needs to be established. The 'tilted plate' might be helpful (see Joe Church profile p 253 or Simpson, 1999, p 111). Use of a diet diary or recall of a typical day's intake can give information about their usual pattern of eating. Without violating cultural norms, they could be educated on a healthier pattern of eating to reflect their changed needs in later life.

References

Fieldhouse, P. (1995). Food and Nutrition – Customs and Culture. London: Chapman and Hall.

Griep, M.I., Verleye, G., Franck, A.H., et al (1996). Variation in nutrient intake with dental status, age and odour perception. European Journal of Clinical Nutrition 50(12): 816–825.

Norton, B. (1996). Nutritional Assessment. Nursing Times 92(26): 71–76.

Shamash, J. (1998). Haunted memories. Nursing Standard 12(26): 26–27.

Simpson, P. (1999). In: Hogston, R., Simpson, P. (Eds) Foundations of Nursing Practice. Basingstoke: Macmillan. Eating and drinking: pp 93–132.

Webb, G.P., Copeman, J. (1996). The Nutrition of Older Adults. London: Edward Arnold.

Further reading

Carlowe, J. (1998). Orthodox care. Nursing Times 94(48): 32–33.

Palmer Keenan, D. (1994). In the face of diversity: modifying nutrition education delivery to meet the needs of an increasingly multicultural consumer base. Journal of Nutrition Education 28(2): 86–91.

RCN Race and Ethnicity Sub-Committee (1998). Nursing older people from ethnic minority communities (summary). Nursing Standard 12(51): 29–30.

Useful Websites

Arthritis and Rheumatism Council: main arthritis medical research charity in the UK.
www.arc.org.uk
Links to many other arthritis sites.
www.arthritislink.com

£400 million is spent on hospital food (Garrow, 1994) from kitchen departments. Food hygiene regulations ban the storage and preparation of food in ward areas and kitchens.

The existence of hospital-induced malnutrition is now well recognised, but the identification and treatment of elderly people at risk of hospital-induced malnutrition continues to be a problem (Brown, 1991).

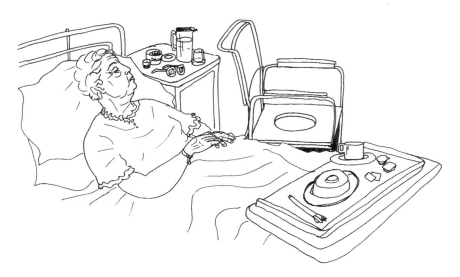

Figure 33.1: Bad practice for eating in hospital.

Answer to question three:
Describe a regimen for healthy eating that may be beneficial to Sabrina whilst she is in hospital.

Thomas (1998) believes that nutritional support to supplement a poor diet, either by mouth or enteral feeding, has improved the likelihood of survival in elderly patients with fractured neck of femur and chest infections.

A regimen for healthy eating whilst in hospital should include the following:

- It is important to establish good hygiene habits for both nurse and patient. Handwashing is often neglected, as is teeth cleaning after a meal
- There also needs to be an adequate fluid intake of at least 1.5 l/day
- Three meals a day, containing all the elements of a balanced diet should be consumed
- 'Snacking' between meals should not be encouraged
- Drinking 1–2 pints of milk per day will provide essential vitamins
- Encourage fresh fruit and salads; peeled and cut up fruit will be easier to manage for some elderly people

---

NB: A balanced diet should contain:

Protein breaks down to provide amino acids, which build and repair body tissue. As Sabrina is not eating well, she will need extra protein in her food.

Fibre comes from foods grown in the ground. Fruits, vegetables, cereal and pulses all contain fibre. Wholemeal products contain more fibre than 'white' products. Although fibre is not a nutrient it is important in a balanced diet. Its bulk keeps the bowel healthy, preventing constipation and other bowel problems.

Vitamins regulate vital functions and assist the body to use food properly.

Carbohydrates are starches and sugars that provide energy.

Fats also supply energy and essential fatty acids. They also assist in the carriage of vitamins.

Minerals build and maintain bones, teeth and blood. They are also vital for the proper functioning of nerves and muscles. To meet daily requirements a wide variety of foods, e.g. low-fat dairy products, green vegetables and wholemeal cereals are needed.

(Adapted from Simpson, 1999)

- Take care of the patient's mouth; make sure the patient's teeth are clean and free from disease
- The patient's individual preferences should be considered as far as food choices are concerned
- Serve small, attractive meals at the correct temperature
- The patient should not be hurried, but allowed to eat the meal in peace and quiet

- Make sure that the patient is correctly positioned to eat (Fig. 33.2) and give encouragement to ask for more.

If food supplements are needed, perhaps an alternative menu could be offered; soups and desserts could be supplemented to increase their protein, vitamin and mineral content. Additional sauces and gravy should be available. Some foods may need to be pureed or liquidised.

Nutritionally complete drinks provide complete and balanced nutrition (Harvey, 1998). Some examples of these are Ensure, Ensure Plus, Freubin, Liquisorb and Fortisip. There are some desserts available that have extra calories for those who may have difficulty with eating. These are Formance and Protipudding.

An overenthusiastic approach to 'feeding' Sabrina may worsen the situation. It may create anxiety or further indifference to food, which will further limit her nutritional intake. Rupert may be anxious about meals and nutrition and so should be included in any plans to help Sabrina regain her appetite and eat a balanced diet.

An adequate nutrient intake is important for maintaining good health. Provided a varied diet is eaten, even in fairly small amounts, nutritional deficiency is not a natural consequence of hospitalisation in elderly people.

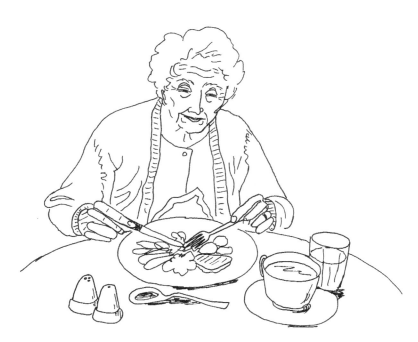

Figure 33.2: Good practice for eating in hospital.

Client profiles in nursing: adults & the elderly

References

Brown, K. (1991). Improving intakes. Nursing Times 87(20): 64–68.

Chu, P. (1998). The nutritional response to trauma in older people. Professional Nurse 13(9): 597–600.

Eastwood, M. (1997). Hospital food. New England Journal of Medicine 336(17): 1261.

English National Board for Nursing, Midwifery & Health Visiting (1995). Nutrition for Life: issues for debate in The Development of Education Programmes. London: English National Board.

Garrow, J. (1994). Starvation in hospital. British Medical Journal 308(6934): 934.

Harvey, J. (1988). Nutrition. In: Tschudin, V. (Ed.) Nursing the Patient with Cancer. Hemel Hempstead: Prentice Hall: pp 107–119.

Holmes, S. (1998). Food for thought. Nursing Standard 12(46): 23–27.

Hunter, M. (1989). Nutrition and the elderly. Nursing Standard 4(2): 38–40.

Robinson, G., Goldstein, M., & Levine, G.M. (1987). Impact of nutritional Status on DRG length of Stay. Journal of Parenteral and Enteral Nutrition 11(1): 49–51.

Simpson, P.M. (1999). Eating and drinking. In: Hogston, R., Simpson, P.M. (Eds) Foundations of Nursing Practice. Basingstoke: Macmillan: pp 93–132.

Thomas, A.J. (1998). Nutrition and the elderly. Nutrition in practice: 10. Nursing Times 94(8): 1–6.

Walters, E. (1998). Know about nutritional assessment. Nursing Times 94(8): 68–69.

Webb, G.P., Coleman, J. (1996). The Nutrition of Older Adults. London: Arnold and Age Concern.

Wood, E.S., Creamer, M. (1996). Malnutrition in hospitals: the nurses' role in prevention. Nursing Times 92(26): 67–70.

Obesity 1

Vivienne Mathews

Esau Fisk is a 71-year-old Londoner, who lives in a converted railway carriage in what can only be described as other peoples' allotments. He has been divorced once, separated from several live-in partners, and now lives in hope that he will marry again. He served in the navy for many years, learning the trade of a chef. Since leaving the navy and his divorce, he has had a succession of jobs, none of which lasted for more than a few years, as his belligerent personality and heavy drinking did not endear him to his employers. He has no children and few friends, finding superficial social contacts in pubs and gambling clubs.

The facilities in his railway carriage home are few: a chemical toilet, which he only empties when overflow levels are reached, no mains gas or electricity and no running water. He relies on an outside cold water tap and on Calor gas for cooking, heat and light. He has been known to run out of gas completely, leaving himself in the cold and dark for several days until his pension is due and can be used to purchase more gas.

Esau Fisk is large; he weighs in excess of 25 stone (160 kg). (The scales in the geriatric day hospital weigh up to 25 stone only, so accurate measurement was not possible!) His mobility is severely compromised; he uses two sticks when walking as osteoarthritis and a degree of heart failure compound his walking ability. His breathing is also a problem, with raised blood pressure and occasional incontinence problems. He has had episodes of small haemorrhages in his mouth over the past few months.

Esau Fisk attended the day hospital as part of a rehabilitation package. He has been moved from his home in order that fumigation and refurbishment can be carried out, and now resides, temporarily, in a rest home which he detests. As he says, it is full of 'old people' amongst whom no kindred spirits are to be found. He treats the nurses with a mixture of highhandedness and sexual innuendo, which the younger carers find difficult to cope with and so tend to avoid him as much as possible.

Question one: What are the dangers of obesity to Esau Fisk's health?
10 minutes

Question two: Summarise the strategies that could be used to encourage Esau Fisk to adopt a positive approach to weight loss.
20 minutes

Question three: Outline the principles of a healthy diet for Esau Fisk.
10 minutes

Time allowance: **40 minutes**

Answer to question one:
What are the dangers of obesity to Esau Fisk's health?

WHO (1998) officially recognises that obesity has reached epidemic proportions. It goes on to say that without successful intervention, the numbers of obese people will double every 10 years. It has been estimated that the direct and indirect effects of obesity cost approximately 5% of the total health care budget of affluent countries (Prentice, 1997).

> **NB:** Obesity is identified by a body mass index (BMI) of >26, which is calculated by dividing weight (kg) by height squared (M).
> (Crombie, 1999)

Obesity has detrimental effects on health, leading to heart disease, stroke, non-insulin-dependent diabetes and cancer. The risk of complications from these conditions increases in line with increased weight. It shortens life expectancy and can exacerbate other problems, such as osteoarthritis (Crombie, 1999).

For Esau Fisk, his deteriorating heart and lungs will contribute to his immobility by causing breathlessness, ankle swelling, chest pain and/or pain in the legs on walking. His obese state will also aggravate these already present difficulties (Prentice, 1995).

It may be that Esau Fisk has a vitamin C deficiency that has come to light following confirmation of the level of ascorbic acid in the white blood cells and platelets in his blood. This would explain the small haemorrhages in his gums and under his tongue. Other problems that are not life threatening, such as osteoarthritis, generalised joint and back pain and some psychological problems will cause a great deal of discomfort and misery for him (Crombie, 1999).

It may be that Esau Fisk has suffered bullying as a child, because of his weight; he may also have experienced social censure and prejudice for most of his adult life in terms of negative opportunities for education, employment and social interaction (Prentice, 1997).

Answer to question two:
Summarise the strategies that could be used to encourage Esau Fisk to adopt a positive approach to weight loss.

Some health care professionals tend to view obesity pessimistically, in terms of the ability to self-manage, so that often the treatment is geared towards specific symptoms, e.g. hypertension, and only minimal attempts are made to tackle the underlying obesity (Hoppe & Ogden, 1997).

People on a low income, such as Esau Fisk, tend to buy cheaper foods that are full of calories and eat them in huge quantities. There is a dilemma of priorities as to whether money is spent on essentials such as fuel and clothing or on beer, burgers, and fish and chips.

Esau (although as a trained chef it might be difficult) has to overcome his unsuitable domestic arrangements for cooking and storing food. Input from an occupational therapist can advise on alterations and cooking skills.

Meals on wheels and luncheon clubs take great care over the nutritional content of their meals, so perhaps this is an avenue that Esau Fisk could approach for his main meal of the day.

It may be that Esau, along with a lot of British people aged over 65 or older, does not have his own teeth. His dentures may be ill fitting and the cost of a new set prohibitive. Taste sensation and salivary flow decreases with age, which will prevent Esau from eating foods other than easily prepared, softish commodities that will be of nutritional value to him (Bond, Coleman & Peace, 1993).

Moderate weight loss, 10% of body weight for example, will improve Esau Fisk's general health. It has been shown that for some people, a return to their ideal body weight is impossible to achieve and that some people, such as Esau Fisk, will be unable to continue to lose weight for longer than 12–16 weeks (SIGN, 1996). Therefore, to encourage Esau Fisk to start a diet that he will have to follow for the rest of his life, could be seen as unrealistic. Weight loss should be aimed at a moderate level of 1 kg per week, over a period of 3 months, followed by long-term maintenance of that loss (SIGN, 1996).

Esau Fisk should be well motivated – to get out of the rest home at least – and amenable to advice! Even if he does not want to lose weight or feels that he cannot, he should be counselled against further gains in weight with the offer of support should he change his mind (Crombie, 1999). He should be advised that he will not undo years of overeating in a few short months nor to have unrealistic expectations of himself that will result in failure and distress.

Ideally, Esau Fisk should adopt a high-carbohydrate, low-fat diet, but will find that terms such as 'reduce', 'cut out', 'avoid' or 'eat less of' deliver a negative message. Kirk (1997) states that increasing intake of carbohydrates alone will reduce fat intake. This indicates a positive response to a diet and by increasing carbohydrates to provide 55% of his total energy intake Esau Fisk will be able to eat:

- Bread
- Potatoes
- Cereals

- Vegetables
- Pastas
- Rice
- Pulses
- Grains.

Couple this with five portions of vegetables and fruit spread throughout the day and, in moderation, some sugary foods such as jam, low-fat yoghurts, puddings and sweet biscuits, Esau Fisk may find a dietary regimen that will encourage normal eating patterns that he can stick to.

Physical activity is crucial in any weight loss programme as a sedentary lifestyle combined with fat and energy-laden fast foods, as in Esau Fisk's present diet, creates a perfect environment in which to gain weight. He should be encouraged to:

- Walk for a minimum of 20 minutes per day, 5 days per week. He should take it gently at first, building up to this level as and when he can
- Limit television watching and therefore 'snacking'
- Get active about the house (or railway carriage in his case): clean up, empty the toilet when it should be done, tidy things away, garden, do his washing, ironing and take time to prepare fresh fruit and vegetables for himself
- Keep motivated by involving friends
- Take it gently, so that disillusionment is kept away.

NB: Esau Fisk may be anxious about how he looks (after all he does want to get married again!) so clinging sportswear and vigorous callisthenics will not be his cup of tea.

Limitations of size, fitness levels and social circumstances should be taken into account.

Answer to question two:
Suggest and justify specific helpful food choices, preparation and lifestyle changes Fiona needs to make.

A BMI of 30 is clinically obese (Thomas, 1998). The energy expended must be balanced by the energy gained. In Fiona's case, her energy intake must be less than her energy output in order to lose weight. She generally needs to be more active (Legge, 1998) – to exercise for 30 minutes five times a week and to eat less. Her requirements will be of the order of 2110 kilocalories (kcal) per day. Many measures are now quoted in kilojoules (kJ), of which there are 4.186 to the kcal.

Obesity will reduce her life expectancy, the increased weight affecting related conditions such as coronary heart disease, diabetes, gallstones, hypertension, lipid abnormalities, osteoarthritis and respiratory disease, not to mention endometrial and large bowel malignancies. She may well experience psychological and social problems as well (Carlisle, 1998; Thomas, 1998).

Fiona needs to know which foods are calorie-dense so that she can eat them with caution.

- Fat – 9 kcal/37 kJ per gram
- Alcohol – 7 kcal/29 kJ per gram
- Carbohydrate – 4 kcal/16 kJ per gram
- Protein – 4 kcal/17 kJ per gram

(Simpson, 1999)

As she works in a supermarket, she may well have access to cheap or discounted foods and excellent leaflets about food, and there may be one on losing weight. She should have written information and support from the practice nurse, who may arrange for her to join a group or an 'exercise prescription' for a local fitness centre, swimming pool, or walking group. It is essential for her short- and long-term health that she becomes more active (Barasi, 1997), as well as eating more healthily. The key is to find an activity that she enjoys, such as bowling, line dancing, clubbing or roller blading.

The distribution of food across the day may affect how many calories are absorbed. Breakfast 'kick-starts' the metabolism; the main meal of the day should be lunch, and the evening meal a light one. 'Loading' the calories at the end of the day means that there is little chance to burn them off. The role of exercise cannot be ignored in terms of enhancement of mood as well as burning more calories. The changes made should be part of lifestyle modification, not 'going on a diet'. Diets do not work; eating sensibly does. 'Yo-yo' dieting tends to replace fat removed from the hips with fat around the waist, transforming her from a 'pear' to an 'apple' shape, which increases her risk of coronary heart disease.

The best weight loss is a slow one of no more than 1 kg/week (2.2 lb), especially as Fiona may not have finished growing upwards. If her activity levels are being increased markedly, the weight loss could and should be slower, as muscle is heavier than fat. A pound of muscle is the size of a bar of soap; a pound of fat, the size of a football. Muscle is more metabolically active tissue and more useful to general health, rendering its owner more resilient.

Client profiles in nursing: adults & the elderly

References

Barasi, M.E. (1997). Human Nutrition: A Health Perspective. London: Arnold.

Legge, A. (1998). Cut the fat. Nursing Times 94(14): 28–29.

Carlisle, D. (1998). The big issue. Nursing Times 94(14): 26–27.

Simpson, P.M. (1999). Eating and drinking. In: Hogston, R., Simpson, P.M. (Eds) Foundations of Nursing Practice. Basingstoke: Macmillan: pp 93–132.

Thomas, D. (1998). Managing obesity: the nutritional aspects. Nursing Standard 12(18): 49–55.

Further reading

Grace, C. (1998). Nutrition and weight reduction. Nursing Times (Suppl 94(24): S1–S6.

Johnson, W.G., Hinkle, L.K., Carr, R.E. et al. (1997). Dietary and exercise interventions for juvenile obesity: long-term effects of behavioural and public health models. Obesity Research 5(3): 257–261.

Thompson, S.B.N. (1993). Eating Disorders: A Guide For Health Professionals. London: Chapman & Hall.

Useful Websites

Rating menus of major fast food outlets www.bgsm.edu/nutrition/FFMainF.htm (Accessed 2000, April 17).

Gives a wide range of options, including calorie charts www.healthnet.org.uk (Accessed 2000, April 17).

Osteoporosis

Vivienne Mathews

'I'm worried about Polly! She's just come back from a holiday in Malaga with a broken wrist. Apparently, it happened when she was getting off the bus taking them to their hotel from the airport. What a start to the holiday! Mind you, its not the first time something like this has happened. Seven months ago, or thereabouts, she broke her ankle and that was only tripping over the hose pipe in the garden. Before that, it was her left arm when she was playing football with the children.

'The trouble is, that I've had osteoporosis for most of my adult life. This means that I've been in pain since the menopause and that would be about 20 years ago. And I think she's got it!

'Well, my sister, Polly's mother, had it and she died 2 years ago after a long stay in hospital with, first, a fractured pelvis (How she did that I'll never know!) and then a fractured hip 6 months later. They told us she had some sort of complications following the surgery, thrombosis, I think!

'Now me, I'd been in good health for some time; taken no pills or anything. I still like a cigarette now and then, but not regularly, if you know what I mean. I finished with periods at the age of 49. As there were no horrid symptoms, not even one hot flush, I didn't take HRT. Well, it wasn't very well known then, and people talked about a link with breast cancer and I didn't want that, but no one told me of its advantages, so I didn't bother to take it.

'Anyway, I fractured my wrist first of all – just like Polly now – then had excruciating pain in my back. I shrank. Don't laugh, but I used to be 5ft 6in now I'm 5ft 3in. I've broken both hips, at various times, and live with pain all the time.

'Polly is only 44 and she's got it, I'm sure! Thank God, I had four sons'.

Question one: What is osteoporosis and what are its most commonly seen effects?

15 minutes

Question two: What are the advantages and disadvantages for Polly of taking HRT?

15 minutes

Question three: Outline the treatment that Polly may be given if osteoporosis is diagnosed.

15 minutes

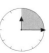

Time allowance: **45 minutes**

Client profiles in nursing: adults & the elderly

Answer to question one:
What is osteoporosis and what are its most commonly seen effects?

Osteoporosis is a disease that is characterised by excessive bone loss, low bone mass and deterioration of bone-making tissue, so that bones become fragile and are susceptible to fracture (Martin, 1998).

The term 'osteoporosis' means porous bone. It is a major health care issue affecting the independence and quality of life of thousands of people. In fact, in the UK 60 000 hip fractures, 40 000 vertebral fractures and 50 000 other fractures occur each year as a direct result of osteoporosis in postmenopausal women. It costs the NHS an estimated £750 million a year (National Osteoporosis Society, 1995).

Osteoporosis affects 1:4 women over the age of 70. There are currently 2 million women with osteoporosis, who have a steadily decreasing quality of life through deformity and pain (Dover, 1994).

> **NB:** Marguerite thanks her lucky stars that she has sons and no daughters, clearly implying that she believes men do not inherit the condition. This is not so! Men do suffer from osteoporosis but not to the same extent. For example, 1:22 men have brittle or porous bones. Between the ages of 70 and 80, 1:40 men will have sustained an osteoporosis-related fracture.
>
> (Holmes, 1998)

The bones of the skeleton are constantly being regenerated through remodelling. This is a process where bone is eliminated by specialist osteoclast cells (resorption). Simultaneously, deposits of new bone (formation) from osteoblast cells, replace the destroyed bone. Problems arise when resorption removes bone faster than formation can replace it. Bone density is then diminished and osteoporosis is the result. Fractures occur in all parts of the skeleton as bone mass recedes, e.g. vertebral crush fractures, Colles fractures of the radius and fractures of the proximal femur (Girvin, 1998).

> **NB:** Bone mass: Peak bone mass is reached at about the age of 40, after which bone loss occurs in both men and women. Women encounter accelerated bone loss so that by the age of 70 they have lost 50% of their bone mass; while men, by the age of 90 have lost just 25% of their higher peak bone mass.
>
> (Martin, 1998)

Although osteoporosis is a condition affecting most elderly people, the foundations are laid in earlier life, through lifestyle and genes.

The risk factors for osteoporosis include:

- Family history of osteoporosis, especially hip fractures in female relations
- Being female
- Being over 50 years of age
- Having an early menopause or hysterectomy (reduced levels of oestrogen cause a lower bone mass, particularly in the spine)
- Immobility or lack of exercise over a long period
- Smoking or drinking heavily (smoking causes low oestrogen levels and alcohol prevents calcium absorption)
- A chronic low intake of calcium in the diet
- Insufficient exposure to sunshine
- Being overly thin; suffering from anorexia nervosa or bulimia (some elderly women in institutional care also suffer bone loss through vitamin D deficiency)
- Women who have lots of missed periods for whatever reason
- Chronic liver, kidney and digestive diseases
- Women who have overexercised, e.g. marathon runners (these women have amenorrhoea because of the over harsh treatment their bodies are taking)
- Patients receiving corticosteroid treatment
- People who have lost several inches in height
- Women who have never borne a child.

(Adapted from Dover, 1994)

Vertebral fractures cause a lot of pain. This is because crush fractures (Fig. 36.1) have healed badly, resulting in distortion and displacement of the spinal vertebrae. When several vertebrae have collapsed they become wedge-shaped, bending the upper spine, pushing the head and neck forward and downward, thus making the characteristic 'dowager's hump' (Fig. 36.2). In turn, this leads to loss of height because of shortening and compression of the spine. Lung capacity is reduced and the resultant kyphosis interferes with actions of the

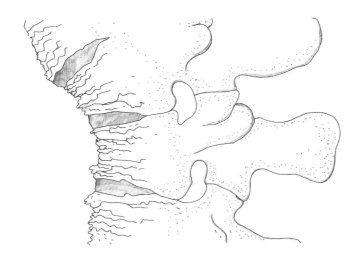

Figure 36.1: Fractures of the spine (crush #) heal badly – over a period of time cause compression fractures which cause the spine to collapse.

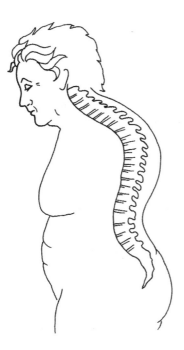

heart, lungs, stomach and bladder. It causes difficulties with breathing and incontinence. It may also cause hiatus hernia (Girvin, 1998). It affects digestive function and leads to back and referred pain. Elderly people may become embarrassed by their physical appearance, as their clothes no longer fit properly and mobility becomes difficult.

Figure 36.2: Osteoporotic spine causing stooped posture.

NB: When an elderly person shrinks 3 or 4 in and stoops, their clothes will dip at the front and ride up at the back, whilst gaping at the neck. The abdomen may bulge as a result of osteoporosis, so blouses and skirts may be a better option than a dress; side zips and front buttoning will be easier to manage than zips at the back.

Answer to question two:
What are the advantages and disadvantages for Polly of taking HRT?

Research has shown that HRT prevents excessive bone loss and fractures in post-menopausal women (Loach, 1998). It is effective in restoring oestrogen levels and so treats bone loss. Fleming (1998) suggests that focusing on younger women could be a cost-effective way of preventing osetoporosis in the next generation.

Medical evidence suggests that taking HRT has many benefits:

- Ability to slow bone loss in people with established osteoporosis
- Ability to reduce the risks of fractures, if taken for at least 5 years, starting soon after menopause
- It may help to reduce the risk of coronary heart disease
- HRT relieves menopause symptoms, especially hot flushes, night sweats, tiredness and irritability.

Recently, oestrogen has been linked with an increased risk of endometrial

> **NB:** Women who take HRT have double protection against both coronary heart disease and excess bone loss. Protection against coronary heart disease is afforded by taking medication with similar hormones to those present in women's bodies before the onset of the menopause; HRT restores the hormone levels and is now believed to be the most effective way of preventing coronary heart disease.
>
> (Dover, 1994)

cancer. To counteract this eventuality, HRT preparations include progesterone, which allows the uterus to remove the endometrium by promoting monthly bleeds, thereby reducing the risk of cancer.

There are side-effects associated with HRT therapy:

- Nausea (usually only a temporary condition)
- Breast tenderness (again, this usually disappears)
- Fluid retention
- Slight weight gain
- Swollen ankles

(Steele, McKnight, Gilchrist, Bennet, Taggart, 1997)

Polly may experience all or none of these side-effects, but by asking her GP for advice, the dose of HRT can be adjusted to reduce all side-effects. Most women feel a definite improvement in both menopausal symptoms and their zest for life. Their sex lives improve, they look younger and feel more energetic than they have for years.

Polly, after commencing HRT should have regular checks on her height, weight, BP and breasts.

Men should also be screened for osteoporosis, especially those with low testosterone levels (about 20% of male osteoporosis sufferers). Testosterone replacement therapy does help to reduce bone loss, and there is some research that indicates oestrogen may be helpful for men with osteoporosis (National Osteoporosis Society, 1995).

HRT improves quality of life and may also prolong life for many elderly people, whether it was initiated at menopause or much later (Holmes, 1998).

Answer to question three:
Outline the treatment that Polly may be given if osteoporosis is diagnosed.

There are several types of treatment for osteoporosis that will depend upon the extent and severity of symptoms experienced and the underlying cause.

Bone density measurement is used for diagnosis and to monitor the development of the disease. It is also used to supervise the success of treatment. A bone scan that will measure bone mineral density is the most helpful means of diagnosis, e.g. dual energy X-ray absorptiometry (DEXA) scan. Plain X-rays will detect fractures. The types of scans that are available are as follows:

- Dual energy X-ray absorptiometry (DEXA)
- Single photon absorptiometry (SPA)
- Dual photon absorptiometry (DPA)
- Quantative computed tomography (QCT)
- Ultrasound.

(National Osteoporosis Society, 1995)

Change of lifestyle

Polly may have to make changes in her lifestyle in order to prevent osteoporosis, for example she should:

- Give up/reduce smoking
- Reduce alcohol consumption
- Take up some form of weightbearing exercise, e.g. regular walking
- Reduce weight if needed
- Ensure adequate rest.

> **NB:** There is some doubt as to how exercise improves bone mass, but it is known that the result of 'stressing' bone stimulates osteoblast production to create more new bone, while ostoclast activity is slowed, giving an overall gain in bone mass.
>
> (Dover, 1994)

Dietary changes

Dietary calcium supplements can slow the progress of osteoporosis and reduce the risk of possible fractures. For adults over the age of 65, an increased calcium daily intake of 1500 mg is recommended (Holmes,1998). Polly, at the age of 44, should be taking 700 mg/day of calcium (Girvin, 1998).

Sources of calcium are:

- Milk
- Cheese
- Yoghurt

- Brown bread (not wholemeal)
- Canned fish, e.g. pilchards and sardines
- Nuts such as almonds
- Some mineral waters
- Green vegetables, e.g. spinach, broccoli
- Some fruits, e.g. figs and oranges.

Polly should increase her intake of dietary vitamin D, which is needed for calcium and phosphorus metabolism (Dover, 1994). Vitamin D is also synthesised by the body through the action of sunlight on the skin.

Vitamin D is found in:

- Oily fish, e.g. sardines, mackerel and herrings
- Cod liver oil
- Milk and butter
- Egg yolk
- Breakfast cereals
- Skimmed milk powder
- Margarine.

Medications

The following should be recommended to Polly as regards her medication:

- Increase oestrogen levels with HRT at the onset of menopause
- Calcitonin levels should be increased (calcitonin is a hormone that is produced by the thyroid gland. It stops bone loss by interfering with osteoclasts. It can be given by nasal spray or injections)
- Bisphosphonates are chemicals which inhibit bone loss by sticking to the surface of the bone, which will hinder the action of osteoclasts
- Anabolic steroids can be prescribed for men, but as they build up muscle and bone, this may not be appropriate for Polly as they have a masculinising effect if used for any length of time
- Fluoride can also be used in small doses. This will restore bone density and help to reduce spinal fractures. As there is a very narrow therapeutic perimeter, careful monitoring is needed.

(Adapted from Dover, 1994)

Maintaining fitness

Exercise, such as dancing, walking, cycling, running or riding, which are load-bearing exercises, will stress and stimulate bone. A sensible exercise programme that allows for periods of rest and relaxation will bring general health benefits. As Polly is a busy mother and wife, she will need to be sure of resting before she gets too tired.

Pain relief

Many elderly people who have established osteoporosis suffer severe pain, especially if their spine is fractured or curved in any way. Pain relief should be tailored to meet individual's needs, and includes:

- Analgesics
- Heat pads, hot water and ice packs
- Physiotherapy
- Hydrotherapy (can be used effectively to reduce muscle spasm and tension)
- Transcutaneous electrical nerve stimulation (TENS) equipment (can be fixed to a painful area of the body, where it blocks pain messages, stopping them from reaching the brain)
- Acupuncture
- Relaxation techniques.

(Dover, 1994)

Psychological support – from carers

This helps individuals to maintain motivation by remaining committed to exercise programmes, stop smoking or keep on with the diet. Support may be needed to comply with the HRT regimen. For Polly as she ages, support will be needed to help her cope with an altered body image, where confidence needs to be restored and reassurance given. Joining an osteoporosis society may also give much needed support, as will involvement in social activities. Education of both Polly and her carers will be needed.

A clear, preventative plan should be given to Polly so that effective care, that responds to every stage of her illness, can be given to support and encourage her at all times.

References

Dover, C. (1994). Osteoporosis. London: Ward Lock.
Fleming, J. (1998). Osteoporosis: learning together. Nursing Times 94(7): 58–60.
Girvin, J. (1998). Established osteoporosis. Elderly Care 10(2): 23–26.
Holmes, S. (1998). Osteoporosis. Nursing Times 94(1): 20–23.
Loach, L. (1998). HRT or not HRT? Nursing Times 94(1): 25.
Martin, U. (1998). The role of the specialist in osteoporosis. Nursing Times 94(16): 50–51.
National Osteoporosis Society (1995). Local provision for osteoporosis – Essential Requirements for a Hospital-based Clinical Service in the Health District. Bath: National Osteoporosis Society.
Steele, K., McKnight, A., Gilchrist, C., Bennet, D., Taggart, H. (1997). A general practice trial of health education advice and HRT to prevent bone loss. Health Education Journal 56: 34–41.

Useful addresses

Arthritis & Rheumatism Council
Copeman House
St Mary's Court
Chesterfield
Derbyshire S41 7TO

Arthritis Care
18, Stephenson Way
London NW1 2HD

National Osteoporosis Society
PO Box 10
Radstock
Bath BA3 3YB

Pain: self-treatment with cannabis

Vivienne Mathews

Annie and Flash Harroway were arrested on Saturday, 3 March, 1999, for being in possession of a substantial quantity of cannabis. The drug squad was surprised when a routine drug operation revealed the villains to be pensioners in their 70s.

Annie and Flash live in a terraced house in a 1950s-built housing estate. They have no children, as they spent the post-war years living in caravans, touring the country on motorbikes and living off the land by potato and strawberry picking, or setting up tents at carnivals and pop festivals.

Their lifestyle was relaxed, lacking in formal education and health care, with no responsibilities. Both Annie and Flash admit to smoking cannabis and taking amphetamines during their touring days. Flash still smokes 'roll-ups', 60 per day and drinks 2 or 3 pints of real ale per night in The Green Man their local public house.

Annie gave up smoking 20 years ago, following a severe bout of 'flu and tries to discourage Flash from smoking as it exacerbates his hacking cough. She also likes a drink in The Green Man, downing several glasses of cider per night.

Annie has had glaucoma for 18 months and arthritic changes in her left hip and knee for at least 10 years. It has severely affected her mobility and the continuous pain of both conditions has made her depressed, with suicidal tendencies at times. Flash had a transurethral resection of the prostate gland 27 years ago and some education on the dangers of smoking, which he steadfastly ignored, as he does his cough.

Flash was told of the benefits of cannabis, in terms of pain relief for glaucoma and arthritis, by a friend from the pub. Desperate to relieve his wife's pain, he obtained and grew cannabis for home consumption. As he was a superb gardener he was very successful at this, selling it to friends and acquaintances, to augment his weekly smoke and beer money.

Question one: What is the legal position on the use of cannabis in a medicinal role?

15 minutes

Question two: What is the beneficial role of cannabis in the treatment of chronic pain?

15 minutes

Question three: As the use of cannabis is illegal, what methods of pain management are available for Annie?

15 minutes

Time allowance: **45 minutes**

Answer to question one:
What is the legal position on the use of cannabis in a medicinal role?

Cannabis is derived from the resin of the plant *Cannabis sativa* or *Cannabis indica*, and has become well known for its recreational use and hallucinogenic properties, rather than as a therapeutic medicine (Royal Pharmaceutical Society, 1996). It is a tall, hairy, weedy looking plant that provides fibres for use in textiles and rope making. When it's flower heads and leaves are dried, it is then known as marijuana, while hash is the extracted resin (Campbell, 1999).

In Victorian times, cannabis in alcohol was used for the treatment of epilepsy and muscle spasms. Queen Victoria, it is alleged, used it to repress menstrual pain (Lothe, 1999). Cannabis, once so widely used as a sedative or narcotic agent, can no longer be prescribed in this country without specific permission from the Home Secretary. Unauthorised prescription may result in a doctor being struck off, but in spite of this, the illegal recreational use of cannabis continues.

> **NB:** It is a class B drug under the 1971 Misuse of Drugs Act and a Schedule 1 drug according to the 1985 Use of Drug Regulations.
>
> (Carroll, 1997)

There is a difference between the legalisation of cannabis and the decriminalisation of it. Decriminalisation of cannabis use means that because large numbers of people break the law and use cannabis, it should not be a criminal offence to use it. As cannabis is a schedule 1 drug, it is an illegal substance and cannot be prescribed or made legal.

Other names for cannabis include:

- Indian Hemp
- Ganga
- Marijuana
- Wacky Baccy
- Hashish
- Pot
- Blow
- Weed
- Puff.

Types of cannabis include:

- Skunk
- Purple Haze
- Northern Lights.

Answer to question two:
What is the beneficial role of cannabis in the treatment of chronic pain?

In 1840, cannabis was recommended as an appetite stimulant, muscle relaxant, analgesic, hypnotic and anticonvulsant. It was also used as a remedy for migraine. As alternative drugs became available, cannabis use declined and its 5000-year medical history has largely been forgotten.

Increasing numbers of people have learnt that cannabis can be used to reduce the nausea and vomiting induced by chemotherapy and it has been said to lower intraocular pressure in cases of glaucoma, therefore markedly reducing the pain involved. It is used as a muscle relaxant in spastic conditions and as an appetite stimulant in the treatment of human immunodeficiency virus (HIV) infections. Cannabis can also be used for its pain-relieving properties in cases of phantom limb pain, menstrual cramps and migraine (Grinspoon & Bakalar, 1993).

Nausea, vertigo and gastrointestinal upsets, as well as mild depression, panic attacks and outbursts of aggressive behaviour, are symptomatic of a 'toxic' psychosis caused by sensitivity to ingested cannabis. These adverse reactions are often associated with excessive alcohol consumption but may be attributed to cannabis smoking as well (Luke, 1997). These psychotic episodes last from 6–12 hours, depending on the rate of drug metabolism.

According to the Daily Mail (February 19th, 1998), cannabis is safer than drink and cigarettes and that the amount of cannabis smoked, worldwide, does less harm than do the legal substances of alcohol and tobacco.

Cannabis is the least damaging, or 'softest', drug as it has very little effect on major physiological functions. There has never been a case of lethal overdose of cannabis (Grinspoon & Bakalar, 1993). In spite of the escalating use of many other drugs in the UK, e.g. Ecstasy and amphetamines, its use amongst young people is growing (Robertson et al, 1996).

NB: Cannabis smoke has more tars and other damaging particles than tobacco smoke.

The effects of cannabis are usually felt very quickly, making users feel relaxed, happy, giggly and more aware of music and/or colours. Users may lose their inhibitions. There is often an analgesic and anti-emetic effect. Cannabis use, over a long period of time, makes users feel anxious and paranoid, and have bloodshot eyes, a dry mouth and slowed reflexes. The main risk is linked to the tobacco it is usually smoked with, but it can be ingested when mixed with other foods, e.g. hash cake; in this case, it is hard to know when its effects will be felt or how strong the effect will be. The onset may take as long as 90 minutes.

Cannabis is not very water soluble and is, therefore, absorbed into the fatty tissues, so that for some time after ingesting or smoking it, it diffuses gradually out of adipose tissues and can be detected in the bloodstream. Traces of cannabis can be found in the blood weeks after using it (Campbell, 1999).

The possible medical applications of cannabis include:

- Chemotherapy for treatment in cancer
- Glaucoma
- Multiple sclerosis
- AIDS wasting syndrome
- Chronic pain
- Migraine
- Menstrual pain
- Labour pain
- Spinal injury spasms
- Epilepsy
- Depression and other mood disorders
- Pruritis.

(Adapted from Carroll, 1997)

The Home Office has licenced G. W. Pharmaceuticals to grow cannabis for therapeutic research. Up to 2000 people with multiple sclerosis are expected to take part in the trial to establish whether cannabis has the ability to reduce pain and relieve muscle spasm (Home Office, 1999).

Answer to question one:
Write a definition of Parkinson's disease and describe its signs and symptoms.

In an essay on The Shaking Palsy, James Parkinson recognised and reported on a disorder of movement and posture (Stewart, 1996).

Parkinson's disease is a common, degenerative, neurological disorder affecting the basal ganglia of the brain (Fig. 38.1). There is depletion of the neurotransmitter, dopamine. This lack produces diffuse, neuromuscular symptoms (Burke & Walsh, 1992).

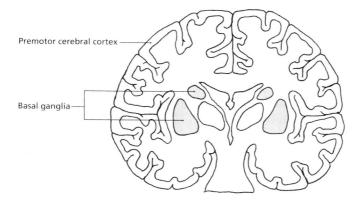

Premotor cerebral cortex

Basal ganglia

Figure 38.1: Brain showing the location of the basal ganglia.

The white matter of the brain contains small, grey areas, known as the basal ganglia. Their primary function is concerned with the control of motor activity descending from the motor cortex. The degeneration that becomes apparent, is in the chemicals produced by the basal ganglia: firstly, dopamine, which has an inhibiting affect on muscle movement and secondly, acetylcholine, a chemical transmitter that stimulates muscle movement. The effect of motor control without the inhibiting influence of dopamine, leads to uncontrollable, rhythmic twitching of groups of muscles, hence the characteristic tremor of Parkinson's disease (MacMahon, 1994).

NB: Parkinson's disease, or paralysis agitans, is an incurable, progressive, degenerative disease. Parkinsonism, on the other hand, is akin to Parkinson's disease but has clinical differences, an absence of tremor, for example. It does not respond to treatment with levadopa; there is an early onset of dementia with abnormalities of eye movements and cerebella ataxia. It is estimated that as many as 1 in 10 people that are diagnosed with Parkinson's disease have, in fact, Parkinsonism.

(Coni, Davison & Webster, 1993)

The signs and symptoms of Parkinson's disease include:

- Rigidity
- Bradykinesia
- Resting tremor
- Weight loss
- Dysarthria
- Depression
- Drooling
- Dysphagia
- Constipation
- Pain
- Impaired postural control
- Shuffling or 'festinating' gait
- Unblinking, expressionless face
- Micrographia (a progressive reduction in size of handwriting)
- Intellectual failure
- Muscle weakness
- Seborrhoeic warts (causing greasy skin).

(Adapted from Coni et al, 1993)

The first symptom to be noticed is usually a tremor in one hand, characteristically a 'pill rolling' type action that is prominent when the patient is at rest; it can be lessened with intention movement, but is greatly increased by emotion. This would appear to be the case with Maggie, who was greatly distressed by her treatment in the rest home. Her tremor had become almost unbearable to her, all stemming from 'petty cruelty' in the home.

Maggie has the characteristic posture of Parkinson's disease (Fig. 38.2), flexed at the neck, hips and knees, with an immobile face and very slow rate of blinking. She uses short, shuffling steps when walking with no arm swing. She may not be able to stop once she has started to move and her feet may appear, at times, to be stuck to the floor.

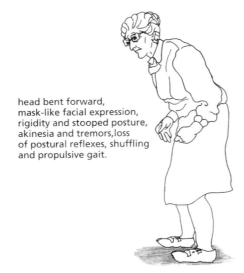

head bent forward,
mask-like facial expression,
rigidity and stooped posture,
akinesia and tremors, loss
of postural reflexes, shuffling
and propulsive gait.

Figure 38.2: Typical Parkinson's posture.

Her unresponsive facial appearance may lead care workers to see Maggie as unfeeling, cold and unattractive, when she is none of these things. Maggie's speech is flat and lacking changes in pitch, tone, inflections and rate (Caird, 1991).

She has lost normal swallowing patterns and there is no lip seal, so that food and saliva drools from her half-open mouth. Food scattering and slow eating will be depressing issues for Maggie.

Features, such as stress, depression and cold temperatures can affect motor performance, so that marked fluctuations are noticed from day to day and throughout each day.

If untreated, Parkinson's disease progresses slowly over a period of many years.

Answer to question two:
Outline the aetiology of Parkinson's disease and explain by the 'on/off' phenomenon.

The prevalence of Parkinson's disease increases with age so that approximately 1 in 1000 people under the age of 60, 5 in 1000 at the age of 70 and 20 in 1000 over the age of 80 will contract the disease (Caird, 1991).

The age of onset is likely to be the late 60s, but 1 in 7 people is diagnosed under the age of 50. Men are slightly more often affected than women. There is no obvious hereditary link for this condition. In all, there are about 60 000 people with Parkinson's disease in the UK (Stewart, 1996).

About 50% of people diagnosed with Parkinson's disease develop dementia (Burke & Walsh, 1992).

The 'on/off' phenomenon is so called because it has been likened, by sufferers, to a light bulb being switched on and off.

The 'off' interval, in which there is no response to drugs is when the patient becomes hypokinetic; some elderly people can predict when an 'off' interval is going to happen, but other people get no warning at all. It is, in these cases, totally unpredictable. The 'on' interval is when drugs are effective and movement is possible. The change from on to off, is abrupt with the patient swinging in and out of control. It is sometimes known as 'yo-yoing' (Caird, 1991).

The length of 'off' intervals can vary from minutes to hours. Care workers can see this as the patient not trying to do things for themselves, after all, 'She could do it yesterday!', which may lead to bad feeling on both sides.

> **NB:** Freezing is a different phenomenon. This occurs without warning and lasts a variable length of time, usually only for a few minutes. The patient, during this time, is unable to complete the motor activity they had started, such as walking, speaking, writing.
>
> (Caird, 1991)

If attempted movement is forced, freezing will be made worse. Any spontaneous action, after a period of distraction, is likely to produce a result in overcoming the freezing phenomenon.

The bent posture of an elderly person with Parkinson's disease means that most of the body weight is pushed forward onto the balls of the feet. They may stand with their heels off the floor, so that initiating movement, with a bent body, flexed knees and precariously balanced on the toes, is very difficult. The centre of gravity should be moved back from the balls of the feet to prompt a more upright posture (Andrews, 1991).

Answer to question three:
How can Maggie be helped to cope with the effects of Parkinson's disease?

The management of Maggie's Parkinson's disease should focus on:

- Maintaining a safe environment
- Supporting communications, both oral and written
- Help with mobility: initiating and maintaining mobility and transfers
- Elimination: control of bladder and bowels; management of constipation
- Medication regimen (see later)
- Nutrition: eating and drinking; swallowing difficulties
- Personal hygiene: washing and dressing
- Psychological problems: depression and confusion
- Establishing sleep patterns; rest and relaxation.

(Stewart, 1996)

Maggie, who is well established on her medication for Parkinson's disease, will know when she needs to take her medication and what doses she should have. She will be very sensitive to small changes in dosages and timing of administration of her medication. Staff in the rest home, who may not be used to a patient with Parkinson's disease, may not fully recognise this and may construe Maggie's repeated requests for her medication as being 'attention seeking' or 'over anxious'.

Drug treatment for Maggie will be aimed at compensating for the dopamine deficiency in the brain. Dopamine, itself, cannot be given orally as it does not pass through the blood–brain barrier. It is usually given as levadopa (L-dopa), which is the precursor of dopamine that does pass from the bloodstream into the brain (Stewart, 1996).

Levadopa improves symptoms related to bradykinesia and rigidity, but is less effective for controlling tremor.

NB: Apomorphine, a dopamine agonist, is used with domperidone (to counteract the side effect of nausea), for people with Parkinson's disease who have severe 'on/off' periods. It works within 10 minutes and the effects last for about 1 hour. Almost all of the patients who have used this drug have experienced severe nausea and vomiting, so it is now given as a subcutaneous injection or a nasal preparation in conjunction with domperidone, an anti-emetic (Maguire, 1997).

Selegiline is relatively free from side-effects, but may cause insomnia or aggravate the side-effects of levadopa. It is used to slow the progress of the disease.

Depression is a feature of Parkinson's disease, but Maggie may have been unhappy, rather than clinically depressed, because of her increased tremor, the effects of decreasing strength in her muscles and her grim living conditions.

Staff in the rest home would benefit from education about Parkinson's disease. They should recognise that adherence to a drug regimen is important, as Maggie may have experienced alterations in functional ability, changing from being active and responsive to being withdrawn and lethargic, in a matter of minutes. Knowing that this is part of the disease progression will help staff to understand some of Maggie's problems and help her to cope with them.

The mental health team should support her anxiety and depression, as well as manage any confusion, delusions, hallucinations or behavioural problems she may have in the late stages of the disease.

Nursing staff will play a significant part in the rehabilitation of Maggie. Initial contact with the patient will help to establish rapport and lines of communication for her; it will allow the nurse to act as a co-ordinator with other members of the multidisciplinary team.

> **NB:** Nurses specialising in the treatment of Parkinson's disease started to appear in 1989. The role has aimed to improve quality of care through the provision of education to other professionals and patients themselves. The families of people with Parkinson's disease also benefit from input and advice on complex drug and care management problems.
>
> (Maguire, 1997)

Disorders of movement are the concern of the physiotherapist, who plays a central role in the treatment of Parkinson's disease. Physiotherapy aims to maintain mobility, maximise function and prevent deformity by concentrating on:

- Increasing and maintaining the range of movement in all joints
- Improving posture and body awareness
- Relaxation
- Gait re-education
- Trunk rotation
- Self-care
- Walking aids
- Compliance
- Functional activities
- Psycho-social state.

Occupational therapy also has an important role to play with patients who have Parkinson's disease. Maggie would benefit from an occupational therapy functional assessment. Advice and support would be given and equipment could be provided to assist in maintaining or increasing independence. Occupational therapy can help Maggie to adjust to her limitations and lead as normal a life as possible within the rest home.

Speech therapy is not required for Maggie, as she is articulate and very vocal. Nevertheless, speech therapy is of enormous value in the treatment of Parkinson's disease, focusing on:

- Respiration
- Phonation
- Articulation
- Prosody – speech hesitation and repetitions
- Voicing
- Lip control
- Tongue control
- Palatal control
- Mastication
- Swallowing.

(Adapted from Caird, 1991)

The dietician could also be involved to encourage a healthy, high-fibre diet, to help manage any possible malnutrition, monitor weight and offer advice to minimise the antagonism of levadopa absorption with protein intake (Maguire, 1997).

A move to a nursing home that provides, or has access to, these services would be the most important step for Maggie to take. Social workers and relatives should provide support and advice throughout the transition time, as by 'voting with her feet' Maggie will be showing her displeasure over the paucity of resources and poor staff attitudes in the rest home, and their imprecise knowledge of Parkinson's disease.

The impact of Parkinson's disease on Maggie has been devastating, but skilled health care professionals can delay severe handicap, improving her quality of life. Using a multidisciplinary approach, Maggie will be enabled to participate in the management of her condition.

References

Andrews, K. (1991). Rehabilitation of the older adult. London: Edward Arnold.

Burke, M.M., Walsh, M.B. (1992). Gerontologic Nursing Care of the Frail Elderly. St Louis, MO: Mosby Year Book.

Caird, F.I. (1991). Rehabilitation in Parkinson's Disease. London: Chapman & Hall.

Coni, N., Davison, W., Webster, S. (1993). Lecture Notes on Geriatrics. (4th ed.). Oxford: Blackwell Scientific Publications.

MacMahon, D.G. (1994). Special report: Parkinson's disease. A paradigm for geriatric medicine. Care of the Elderly 6(4): (Suppl) 51–58.

Maguire, R. (1997). Parkinson's Disease. Professional Nurse 13(1): 33–37.

Stewart, N. (1996). Parkinson's disease: Professional Development Unit No. 24. Nursing Times 92(1): 1–14.

Further reading

Kelly, G. (1995). A self care approach: Parkinson's disease. Nursing Times 91(2): 40–41.

Pinder, P. (1990). The Management of Chronic Illness. London: Macmillan.

Useful addresses

Parkinson's Disease Society
22 Upper Woburn Place
London WC1H 0RA

Carers National Association
29 Chilworth Mews
London W2 3RG

Disabled Living Foundation
380 Harrow Road
London W9

Answer to question three:
What are the main factors necessary for wound healing?

- Protein: necessary for collagen deposition, and lack of it will delay healing and reduce the tensile strength of the wound. White blood cells, needed to combat infection, are manufactured from the protein pool, which if deficient could increase the likelihood of wound infection (Moody, 1995)
- Carbohydrates/glucose: provide the necessary calories for optimal healing; lipids are essential for cell membranes and inflammatory mediators
- Vitamin A requirements are increased by stress or injury, yet vitamin A is considered to increase the inflammatory response, fibroblast differentiation and production of collagen (Olde Damink & Soeters, 1997)
- Vitamin C: an essential co-factor for the synthesis of collagen. A lack of vitamin C will cause a defect in wound healing, failure of collagen synthesis and cross-linking. Joe's previous marginal vitamin C status, coupled with repeated infection and three operations, makes this the most likely cause of his impaired wound healing
- Zinc: essential for fibroblast activity and collagen synthesis, and if deficient, not only will these processes be impaired, but also overall wound strength will be reduced and epithelialisation delayed.

As Joe is malnourished, his wound healing will be prolonged/delayed.

Answer to question four:
What recommendations could be given to maximise Joe's chances of healing completely this time?

A lifestyle assessment to reduce risk factors and enhance healing factors (Simpson, 1998) should be carried out by the surgical nurse or practice nurse. The main features of a healthy diet for Joe to follow during convalescence of approximately 3 months should be outlined in writing in the expectation that some new habits will persist. It may be worth considering multivitamin supplementation to promote wound healing as a cost-effective alternative to losing his job, because of his undergoing the same infection/surgery sequence again. Vitamins must be taken *with* food, which is why they are called supplements.

The 'tilted plate' (Simpson, 1999) system is simplistic, but provides a useful basis against which to measure the weight of food taken, giving a broad indication of balance. It covers not individual meals but whole days or several days. The important thing is that the diet adds up most of the time to 100%. The ideal diet consists of:

1. Starchy foods – 33% – Bread, toast, rolls, breakfast cereals, rice, pasta, noodles, potatoes, chapattis. Joe should consider wholegrain, wholewheat, brown versions of these as they are more filling.
2. Milk and dairy – 14% – Milk, cream, cheese, yoghurt, butter, crème fraîche, ghee (clarified butter – used in foods such as curries). Joe should be taking skimmed milk and low-fat foods.
3. Meat and alternatives – 12% – Meat, poultry, fish, eggs, cooked beans, lentils, cheese. Joe should not need more than 85 g (3 oz) of protein per day when he is well, as the excess will be stored as fat. While he is healing he may need a little more than this.

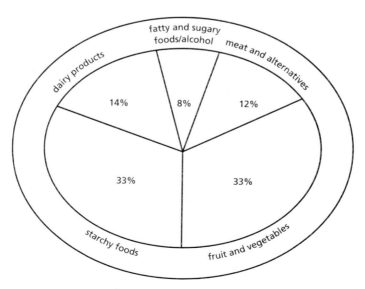

Figure 39.3: The tilted plate (Simpson, 1999).

4. Fruit and vegetables – 33% – Joe needs five different sorts a day to improve his vitamin and mineral intake. They can be fresh, frozen, tinned, dried, or juice. He could consider strategies such as adding tomato to his bacon sandwich, and having orange juice and a piece of fruit with his canteen meal. This will improve his vitamin C status.
5. Fats/oils; fatty foods; sugary foods; alcohol – 8% –

- Fats/oils: Butter, margarine, low fat spread, oil, mayonnaise, oily salad dressing. These are the most calorie-dense foods, so Joe should be cut back on these as much as he can.
- Fatty foods: Fatty meat, luncheon meat, sausages, rich sauces, fatty gravies, cream, cream cheese, ice-cream, pastry, pies, cakes, biscuits, chips, crisps, and packet snacks. These foods may have a lot of hidden fats, and tend to be sources of trans fats, which increase the risk of heart disease. Curries are likely to be high-fat foods.
- Sugary foods: Sugar, honey, jams, marmalade, chocolate, sweets.
- Alcohol: Joe should keep to 21 units or less per week, including two alcohol-free days. He should avoid binging, which does the most harm to health.

Joe should aim to keep his weight steady until the wound has healed, then try to lose a maximum of 1 kg/week (2.2 lb), monitored by the practice nurse if he agrees. Make suggestions of cheap, easy to prepare meals. A range of leaflets are available from most practices, chemists and supermarkets.

Exercise

Joe should increase his activity levels steadily. As healing progresses, the intensity can be increased. At first 20 minutes three times a week, getting warm and breathless is enough, steadily building up to more than 30 minutes, five times a week. At 3 weeks after surgery, the wound is at about 20% of its ultimate strength. Depending on the physical demands of the job, he should consider returning to work. The scar will never be more than 80% of the strength of normal tissue (Olde Damink & Soeters, 1997). He may look at how he travels to work, and consider briskly walking some of the way (see Doris Gaudion profile, p. 67).

Smoking

If Joe has an interest in cutting down or giving up smoking, he needs to be referred to the GP or practice nurse for support. If not, damage limitation techniques suggest an increase in his vitamin C intake as smoking increases excretion and reduces storage of vitamin C.

Alcohol

A unit of alcohol equals a pub measure such as half a pint of ordinary strength beer, lager or cider; a single measure of spirits; or a small glass of wine. By cutting down the alcohol and having more low-calorie soft drinks, Joe may not only reduce his overall calorie intake but also save money.

All information given should be supplied in written form, and targets for his lifestyle changes kept reasonable and manageable. The main objectives for Joe appear to be for his wound to heal, and for him to keep his job. These could be potent motivators for him to persist with his efforts. Joe needs support and encouragement as well as advice.

References

Collier, M. (1996). The principles of optimum wound management. Nursing Times 10(43): 47–52.

Foster, L., Moore, P. (1997) The management of recurrent pilonidal sinus. Nursing Times 93(32): 64–68.

Gould, D. (1997). Pilonidal sinus. Nursing Times 93(32): 59–62.

McVey, M. (1999). Pilonidal sinus: the bottom line. Nursing Times 95(1): 28–29.

Moody, M. (1995). Problem wounds: a nursing challenge. Nursing Standard (RCN nursing update) 9(25): S3–S8.

Olde Damink, S.W.M., Soeters, P.B. (1997). Nutrition and wound healing. Nursing Times supplement: Nutrition in Practice 4: 1–6.

Simpson, P.M. (1998). Introduction To Surgical Nursing. London: Arnold: pp 9–11, 14, 15, 36–42.

Simpson, P.M. (1999). Eating and drinking. In: Hogston, R., Simpson, P.M. (Eds) Foundations of Nursing Practice. Basingstoke: Macmillan: pp 93–132.

Wells, L. (1994). At the front line of care: the importance of nutrition in wound management. Professional Nurse 9(8): 525–530.

Further reading

Chambers, N. (1999). Wound management. In: Hogston, R., Simpson, P.M. (Eds) Foundations of Nursing Practice. Basingstoke: Macmillan: pp 240–266.

Davidson, A. (1995). Surgical infection. Nursing Times 91(39): 59–65.

Hallett, A. (1994). Vital ingredients. Nursing Times 90(50): 64–68.

Men's health magazine.

Ottley, C. (2000). Vitamin and mineral supplements: who needs them? Nursing Standard 14(29): 42–45.

Useful Websites

An interactive website for nutritional information
www.navigator.tufts.edu (Accessed 2000, April 17.)

Pneumonia: health promotion, homelessness in the community

Tinuade Okubadejo

Aliyah John, aged 22 years old, is caring for her boyfriend, Lee Gonzalez, aged 19. Lee is being successfully treated at home by the GP and community nurses for an acute lobar pneumonia caused by infection with *Streptococcus pneumoniae*. Since this was diagnosed early, Lee has not been admitted to hospital and is responding well to antibiotic treatment and physiotherapy.

The family are registered as homeless, temporarily living in bed-and-breakfast accommodation found by a social worker. Aliyah's daughter Venetta, aged 3 years, is from a previous relationship; Lee is the father of Ricardo, aged 6 months. They live in one room, with a shared kitchen and bathroom. There is condensation in the room and a large patch of mould, which the landlord promised to attend to 2 months ago. Both Venetta and Ricardo have 'wheezy' chests; Venetta has been diagnosed with asthma, for which she uses an inhaler.

Aliyah was found to be anaemic after giving birth to Ricardo and although improving, this problem has not resolved.

Aliyah and her boyfriend have been in local authority foster care or residential care almost all their lives for reasons of abuse and neglect, and neither are working. Neither have any academic qualifications, partly due to the experience of constantly moving between foster families and residential homes during their school years. They have no contact with their families, but Lee keeps in contact with a black Pentecostal minister who helped him a great deal when he was a child. This man and his wife have become surrogate parents over the years and the whole church has been supportive by supplying clothes, toys and equipment for the children. Additionally, babysitters and meals are forthcoming. Aliyah, Lee and the children usually see this family weekly. Aliyah utilises the services of a local authority-run drop-in centre for homeless families, where she can do her washing, keep the children warm in the winter and have some time to herself whilst they are cared for in a crèche. She also uses various voluntary services around the area.

The drop-in centre has an attached social worker, health visitor and GP. Aliyah and her family suffer continuously from minor illnesses in addition to the problems previously stated, therefore these services are greatly appreciated.

The whole family relies on benefit payments at present; however, Lee is enrolled on a full-time vocational course at a local college of further education and the fees are paid for him. Aliyah has been attending evening classes for a GNVQ once a week at the same college; her fees are also paid for her. Lee hopes to find a job when he has completed his course and Aliyah intends to find work when Ricardo is 1 year old.

Aliyah and Lee both miss meals on a regular basis; to save money, but they ensure the children are well fed. They have no savings and do not possess a car.

Neither parent has much knowledge about healthy living or the human body; however they are intelligent, motivated to improve their situation and eager to learn. Their priorities are: rehousing, to finish education and find work, and to improve health, particularly through cheap, balanced nutrition. Aliyah is a black British woman; Lee is of mixed racial origins.

Consider the following questions carefully and formulate your answers before turning the page.

Question one: Define pneumonia.

5 minutes

Question two: Compare and contrast the two most common forms of pneumonia: lobar pneumonia and bronchopneumonia.

10 minutes

Question three: How should Lee's illness be treated?

10 minutes

Question four: What are the signs of anaemia in a black person?

5 minutes

Question five: This family belongs to the 'underclass'. Explain the links between serious deprivation and poor health. Which determinants of health are relevant to this case?

15 minutes

Question six: Explore the health promotion issues for this family and postulate some solutions for these. Would their ethnic background have any effect on the solutions?

10 minutes

Question seven: Which agencies could collaborate to improve the situation for this family in the long term?

5 minutes

Time allowance: **1 hour**

Answer to question one:
Define pneumonia.

Pneumonia is an inflammation of the lung parenchyma, in which alveolar air is replaced by a watery inflammatory, protein-rich exudate (James & Studdy, 1993). It is most commonly the result of an infection, and may be primary or secondary in nature (primary pneumonia occurs in an otherwise healthy person; secondary pneumonia results in an individual who is immunosuppressed) (Underwood, 1996).

Answer to question two:
Compare and contrast the two most common forms of pneumonia: lobar pneumonia and bronchopneumonia.

Lobar pneumonia

This pattern of pneumonia is caused by exudate spreading through the alveoli to either a large part of or an entire lobe of the lung, replacing air with fluid.

Signs and symptoms include onset of the following difficulties over several hours: a fever (which may be more than 40°C, with uncontrollable shivering or rigors), a dry cough and the eventual production of sputum, which is pink and sticky initially, becoming purulent and flecked with blood ('rusty') as the disease progresses. Acute chest pain results from deep inspiration (James & Studdy, 1993; Underwood, 1996).

Lobar pneumonia typically affects otherwise healthy adults, more commonly men, in the 20–50 year age group and is uncommon in infants and older people. The vast majority of cases are due to the Gram-positive bacterium *Streptococcus pneumoniae* (Stevens & Lowe, 1995; Underwood, 1996).

Bronchopneumonia (James & Studdy, 1993; Stevens & Lowe, 1995; Underwood, 1996)

This involves inflammation of the terminal and respiratory bronchioles, in a patchy distribution normally affecting basal areas in both lungs simultaneously.

Signs and symptoms are normally: crepitations (crackles) audible with auscultation, fever and a progression to septicaemia and reduced consciousness.

This type of pneumonia more commonly affects elderly people, infants or those with a pre-existing debilitating disease (such as cerebrovascular accident, cancer, acute and chronic respiratory disease). It may also be a complicating factor in patients post-surgery if respiratory secretions are not cleared.

Answer to question three:
How should Lee's illness be treated?

Lobar pneumonia due to *S. pneumoniae* is easily treated with a penicillin-based antibiotic (such as Benzylpen G, amoxycillin, cephalosporin or erythromycin). It tends to respond within a 24-hour time period in a healthy individual (James & Studdy, 1993). If left untreated, it will generally resolve within 8–10 days.

Answer to question four:
What are the signs of anaemia in a black person?

As with white people, the affected individual will feel exhausted, light-headed and dizzy at times. They will have an accelerated pulse rate and tachycardia. The main difference is that anaemia is best observed by checking mucous membranes (inside the mouth or eyelid) since these will look unusually pale rather than a healthy dark pink. Also, black skin loses its normal sheen when an individual is suffering from anaemia, appearing dull and dry.

Answer to question five:
Explain the links between deprivation and illness. Which determinants of health are relevant?

There are many determinants of health; these are factors that affect an individual's health, either positively or negatively (Ewles & Simnett, 1992, pp 3–18). They may be due to genetic, lifestyle, environmental or social factors or to infectious diseases (Naidoo & Wills, 1994). Some of these risk factors can be altered by individual behaviour, e.g. eating a more balanced diet, taking regular exercise, and learning how to deal with minor illness appropriately. Others are fixed and are beyond the ability of an individual to alter, e.g. genetic or environmental factors affecting health, and access to health care, which depend on the area one lives in. Living in poverty has a major impact on health; a wealth of research has established that mortality and morbidity rates are associated with financial income and socio-economic stress levels (Bunton et al, 1995; Bury, 1997; Naidoo & Wills, 1994). Helvie (1998) states that homeless people are more likely to suffer from higher rates of illness than the general population. Chronic illnesses of particular concern include:

- Untreated respiratory tract infections and resulting disorders
- Hypertension
- Arthritis
- Dental infections and problems
- Gastrointestinal disorders and nutritional deficiencies
- Vascular disease
- Neurological disorders
- Eye disorders
- Genitourinary problems
- Musculoskeletal difficulties
- Ear disorders
- Skin conditions.

Acute problems include:

- High rates of trauma
- Respiratory infections
- Skin infections.

It will be extremely difficult for Aliyah and Lee to improve their health until they improve their material circumstances, which at present is beyond their control (Gastrell & Edwards, 1996; Helvie, 1998; Phillips & Verhasselt, 1994). For example, the overcrowded conditions in which they live mean that it is more likely that they will suffer from minor illnesses caused by droplet spread, because they are in closer proximity than a family with more living space, where everyone has their own bedroom. The presence of untreated mould is likely to exacerbate the children's respiratory difficulties, as spores may be released, which are then inhaled and cause an allergic response (Wilkinson, 1996, p 177). The fact that the parents are missing meals and are stressed more than the average parent means they are more likely to be immunosuppressed and therefore prone to the illnesses mentioned earlier (Wilkinson, 1996, p 176).

Lee's recent episode of pneumonia and Aliyah's chronic anaemia are two examples of this immunosuppression.

Traumatic accidents to small children are also more likely in an overcrowded environment, lacking safety equipment and play areas. *The Health of the Nation Key Area Handbook on Accidents*, states that up to the age of 4, most fatal accidents occur in the home, whereas after the age of 5, road traffic accidents are the major cause of accidental fatalities (Department of Health, 1993), possibly due to children playing in or around roads.

There are also psychological or emotional effects from living with such stress (Sandall, 1993), which are likely to strain a relationship to breaking point. The fact that Aliyah and Lee are attempting to remain positive, have some strong social support networks via their church links and are trying, via education, to improve their prospects may give them some protection against this stress and assist them to cope (Helvie, 1998; Wilkinson, 1996).

Their situation is fairly typical for care leavers, of whom 75% have no qualifications and 80% are unemployed (Eaton, 1998). Visible ethnic minorities are also over-represented in the numbers of homeless people (Helvie, 1998).

Answer to question six:
Explore the health promotion issues present for this family and postulate some solutions for these. Would their ethnic background have any effect on the solutions?

Any health care worker attempting to provide support for this family will need to demonstrate a great deal of sensitivity in understanding how difficult their situation is and how intractable and long term their problems may be. Nurses will need to be prepared to learn from their clients how they survive in this situation and which issues they consider priorities. They will also need to work very closely with other agencies, to ensure a coordinated approach of which the young couple feel in control.

The health promotion issues for this family are:

- Increasing disposable income
- Increasing levels of social support
- Dealing with discrimination and racial harassment
- More suitable housing
- Knowledge of how to recognise serious illness
- Knowledge of recognising and treating minor illnesses
- Access to health care
- Increased knowledge about healthy living
- Obtaining balanced nutrition under financial stress
- Obtaining regular exercise.

Increasing disposable income

An increase in disposable income will aid the ability to make choices about healthy living and will improve the health of this family more than any other single item (Bury, 1997).

The nurse needs to encourage both partners to ensure that they are receiving all the benefits that they are entitled to for themselves and the children (Sandall, 1993). More disposable income would permit more frequent washing of bed linen, and the purchase of non-allergenic bed linen, which would help with Venetta's asthma. Similarly the chronic anaemia which Aliyah suffers from could be alleviated if she possessed a larger income to spend on food.

It may be possible, depending upon the opportunities available in their local area, once Aliyah and Lee have completed their courses, have improved curricula vitae and some experience behind them, to obtain work that takes them above benefit levels of income. They need good careers advice at this point in time.

Increasing levels of social support

Wilkinson (1996) gives numerous examples of research suggesting that high levels of social support protect individuals against disease. Nurses need to be aware of the potential health risks of isolation in addition to material stress (Taylor, 1993) and to give clients this information, discussing the importance of building up protective social networks.

Lee and Aliyah could achieve this by making more use of the networks that they already have, including acquaintances from the day centre, college, evening class in addition to the church. It may be that the pooled resources of the church can offer considerable support to this young family, in terms of a surrogate family structure, of child care, meals and advice that is ethnically appropriate.

Dealing with discrimination and racial harassment (Douglas, 1995; Elliott, 1994)

The link between poor health and material disadvantage is also associated with minority ethnic groups, perhaps because many people in these groups suffer from material disadvantage that may be linked with racism (Douglas, 1995). Examples of this are not gaining employment or promotion because of the colour of their skin, which can lead to having to live in substandard housing, which in turn could lead to the types of respiratory pathologies described in the case study.

In addition to their other problems, Aliyah and Lee may encounter difficulty in accessing information and basic public services due to direct or indirect racial discrimination by those in control of these facilities, including poor quality care and stereotyping by employees (Jewson, 1993). They may also become targets of harassment or violence, particularly if they lack control over where they live. Nurses need to be clear that such activity is a criminal offence and be ready to encourage the passing of information on to the police, housing departments, health managers, medical practitioners and social work departments as appropriate. Alternatively, they could pass this information on themselves if the family would prefer them to do so. Action might then be taken to attempt to stop this source of stress; however it may be a lengthy process. It is important for the young parents to be able to discuss these issues with someone who understands their concerns, whether a lay person, a volunteer or an employee of a statutory agency. In their case, someone from the church might possess the necessary skills and resources to advise them. Nurses must be aware of any special groups in their area that may be able to provide support and pass on the details to those clients who are interested. Additionally, they must examine their own practice to ensure that it is free of discriminatory attitudes, including the assumption that Aliyah and Lee must conform to any cultural 'norm' (such as the food they consume).

More suitable housing (Sandall, 1993)

This is a major factor in the improvement of the children's chest conditions and it links with points made in the previous paragraph. Less overcrowding, a home free from damp and a warm environment in winter, will reduce the likelihood of minor coughs and colds, acute asthma attacks and more serious chest infections (Wilkinson, 1996). The nurse should encourage Lee and Aliyah to apply for low-cost housing, bearing in mind that some geographical areas may not be safe for them to live in due to racial harassment.

Knowledge of how to recognise serious illnesses (Renfrew, 1993)

This links in with the previous paragraph on suitable housing. Aliyah and Lee need to be clear about the point at which a minor illness becomes serious and when to seek health advice or medical assistance. Any nurse involved with the family needs to ensure that they are clear about their role in managing Venetta's asthma, particularly the effective delivery of prescribed medication and knowing when to fetch medical help. If necessary, appropriate referrals should be made to the nurse and GP who are managing Venetta's asthma.

Knowledge of recognising and treating minor illnesses (Renfrew, 1993)

If the parents have better knowledge of health promotion and human physiology, they will be better able to care for themselves and for their children and to manage minor illnesses at home safely. The nurses involved with the family should take the time to give basic education in order to facilitate a clear understanding of how health problems arise and can be prevented. This may include the use of appropriate audio-visual material in the course of visits.

Access to health care (Sandall, 1993)

This family should be entitled to some assistance with financial outlay because they are receiving certain types of benefit and have no savings. For example, they should receive free prescriptions, dental treatment and transport costs to appointments. They are fortunate to be registered with a GP, because many homeless families are not accepted onto surgery lists (Sandall, 1993). However, since the practice population tends to be larger in more deprived areas, initial access to appointments is more difficult due to longer waits to see a doctor, than in more affluent areas and the quality of service provision may be worse (Jewson, 1993).

Increased knowledge about healthy living (Renfrew, 1993)

Healthy living is the foundation upon which health is built and will protect against illness occurring in the first place. For example, links between a healthy diet and the reduced likelihood of infectious illness and gastrointestinal cancers are well known. This family will have much more than the average level of difficulty in adopting a healthy lifestyle (Sandall, 1993), but should be encouraged to control the items that they do have power over. Nurses involved with this family should ensure that they are taught about this link, in a practical, non-patronising manner.

Obtaining balanced nutrition under financial stress

It is common for low income parents to miss meals in order to be able to afford other items such as new shoes for children. Part of the problem for the 'under-class' is that cheap, healthy food is more easily obtainable in supermarkets located away from areas in which they live, requiring expensive travel. Additionally, more fresh food, such as fruit and vegetables, is wasted because it is perishable.

If Aliyah and Lee have friends, they could 'bulk buy' and share out these items. Alternatively, if they have access to a freezer, they could purchase frozen fruit and vegetables, which contain relatively high proportions of vitamins and minerals.

Aliyah needs information about relatively cheap sources of iron (such as in dark green leafy vegetables) to combat her anaemia.

Obtaining regular exercise

It will require some thought and determination to find low-cost forms of exercise, particularly with the children in mind. The best means of obtaining exercise for someone on a very low income is probably by walking; but attention needs to be paid to the locality, speed and frequency with which this is done. For example, it is obviously not advisable to walk in an area that is highly polluted by traffic or in a dangerous locality. Walking should be at a speed that induces light perspiration but enables talking. It is best to walk daily, for a minimum of 20 minutes. Alternatively, there may be some low cost or 'prescription' schemes available in council-run leisure centres where GP referral is required (Sandall, 1993). It is possible that the minister's wife could care for the children whilst the young parents exercise.

Finally, the nurse should bear in mind the likelihood that this couple walk much further than the recommended minimum in order to save money and assess this accurately prior to recommending any extra activity.

Answer to question seven:
Which agencies could collaborate to improve the situation for this family in the long term?

- Health professionals
- Social services
- Social support networks (the church; friends)
- Independant voluntary groups (e.g. Shelter; Citizen's Advice Bureau; playgroups)
- Housing agencies dealing with low-cost housing
- Benefits Agency
- Colleges of Further Education and Community Colleges.

References

Bunton, R., Nettleton, S., Burrows, R. (Eds). (1995). The Sociology of Health Promotion, Critical Analyses of Consumption, Lifestyle and Risk. London & New York: Routledge.

Bury, M. (1997). Health and Illness in a Changing Society. London and New York: Routledge.

Department of Health (1993). The Health of the Nation, Key Area Handbook, Accidents. London: HMSO.

Douglas, J. (1995). Developing anti-racist health promotion strategies. In: Bunton, R., Nettleton, S., Burrows, B. (Eds) The Sociology of Health Promotion, Critical Analyses of Consumption, Lifestyle and Risk. London & New York: Routledge: pp 70–77.

Eaton, L. (1998, May 6). Outside chance. The Guardian Newspaper.

Elliott, K. (1994). Working with black and minority ethnic groups. In: Webb, P. (Ed.) Health Promotion and Patient Education. London: Chapman & Hall: pp 195–213.

Ewles, L., Simnett, I. (1992). Promoting Health, A Practical Guide. (2nd ed.). London: Scutari Press.

Gastrell, P., Edwards, J. (1996). Community Health Nursing, Frameworks for Practice. London: Baillière Tindall.

Helvie, C.O. (1998). Advanced Practice Nursing in the Community. London: Sage Publications Inc: pp 128–159.

James, D.G., Studdy, P.R. (1993). A Colour Atlas of Respiratory Disease. (2nd ed.). London: Wolfe Publishing.

Jewson, N. (1993). Inequalities and differences in Health. In: Taylor, S., Field, D. (Eds) Sociology of Health and Health Care, An Introduction for Nurses. Oxford: Blackwell Scientific Publications: pp 57–76.

Naidoo, J., Wills, J. (1994). Health Promotion, Foundations for Practice. London: Baillière Tindall.

Phillips, D.R., Verhasselt, Y. (Eds) (1994). Health and Development. London: Routledge: pp 24–25.

Renfrew, M. (1993). Towards healthier families. In: Wilson-Barnet, J., Macleod Clark, J. Research in Health Promotion and Nursing. Basingstoke: The MacMillan Press: pp 160–173.

Sandall, J. (1993). Homeless families, a Health Promotion challenge. In: Dines, A., Cribb, A. (Eds) Health Promotion concepts and practice. Oxford: Blackwell Scientific Publications: pp 158–173.

Stevens, A., Lowe, J. (1995). Pathology. London: Mosby.

Taylor, S. (1993). Social integration, social support and health. In: Taylor, S., Field, D. (Eds) Sociology of Health and Health Care, An Introduction for Nurses. Oxford: Blackwell Scientific Publications: pp 77–93.

Underwood, J.C.E. (Ed.) (1996). General and Systematic Pathology. (2nd ed.) Edinburgh: Churchill Livingstone.

Wilkinson, R.G. (1996). Unhealthy Societies; the Afflictions of Inequality. London: Routledge: pp 175–192.

Further reading

Naidoo, J., Wills, J. (1994). Health Promotion, Foundations for Practice. London: Baillière Tindall.
Swanson, J.A., Nies, M.A. (1997). Community Health Nursing, Promoting the Health of Aggregates. (2nd ed.). London: W.B. Saunders Company.
Wilkinson, R.G. (1996). Unhealthy Societies, the Afflictions of Inequality. London: Routledge.

Pressure sores, wound healing

Vivienne Mathews

Fred Salisbury is an 83-year-old, retired accountant. He is 1.85 m in height and weighs only 64 kg. He lives with his 80-year-old wife, Bella, in a smart block of flats belonging to a Housing Association. Bella is now rather frail and is dependent on Fred for all activities of living. He remained in good health until he had a stroke that necessitated hospital admission and left him with a severe hemiparesis.

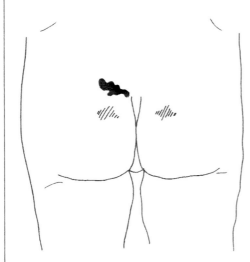

Figure 41.1 Pressure sores.

He was admitted to an acute elderly medicine ward, where it was found that he had profound weakness in his left arm and leg; he was incontinent of urine. As the urinary incontinence continued, he was catheterised.

Two days after admission, redness was noted on his sacrum and, although recorded in a care plan, no action was taken. On transfer to a long-stay ward, some 2 weeks later, it was noted that he had two superficial broken areas of skin, on either side of his buttocks, and a deep suppurating wound leading from the left side towards his sacrum (Fig. 41.1).

Question one: Discuss the factors that may influence the development of pressure sores.

15 minutes

Question two: Contrast the effects of pressure, shear and friction on the skin of an elderly person.

15 minutes

Question three: How should the risk of Mr Salisbury developing a pressure sore have been assessed, and what steps should have been taken to prevent this from happening?

15 minutes

Time allowance: **45 minutes**

Answer to question one:
Discuss the factors that may influence the development of pressure sores.

Pressure sores are common in elderly care settings because of elderly peoples' high-risk status (Timmons, 1999).

Causes of pressure sores

Mechanical forces include:
- Pressure
- Shear
- Friction
- Poor patient handling.

Reduced tissue tolerance is caused by:
- Poor nutrition
- Increased age
- Chronic/acute illness
- Poor oxygen perfusion
- Drugs
- Emaciation
- Poor skin care
- Incontinence.

Reduced mobility is caused by:
- Surgery
- Lowered levels of consciousness
- Drugs
- Illness
- Neurological problems
- Poor muscle strength.

(Adapted from Pendleton, 1998)

Factors that influence the development of pressure sores can be divided into two categories:

1. *Extrinsic factors*:
   - Pressure
   - Shear
   - Friction.

2. *Intrinsic factors*:
   - General health status
   - Immobility
   - Cardiovascular state
   - Nutritional status

- Anaemia
- Incontinence
- Smoking
- Neurological disease
- Infection
- Increased age
- Steroid use
- Sedative use.

There is considerable diversity in individuals' skin type and composition, which are dependent on age, environment and ethnic origin, but dry skin with a water content of less than 10% is common in elderly people (Nathan, 1997).

The skin is relentlessly subjected to mechanical injury so that the cells of the basal layer within the epidermis are continuously renewed. In a period of about 2 weeks, the cells, under pressure from below, rise to the skin's surface in the form of flattened packets of protein. The protein inside these epidermal cells attracts water molecules so that very little water is lost from the skin (Courtenay, 1998).

As a person ages, the epidermis thins and loses its ability to retain moisture; the skin therefore becomes dry. Dry skin is associated with dermatitis and eczema; it is also a factor in the formation of pressure sores. Rehydration of the skin with warm bath water, the application of emollients and emulsions such as aqueous cream, and a gentle patting of the skin until it is dry will sooth and rehydrate the skin, helping to prevent the development of pressure sores (Nathan, 1997).

Answer to question two:
Contrast the effects of pressure, shear and friction on the skin of an elderly person.

These three mechanical forces are the main causes of pressure sores.

1. *Friction*: occurs when two surfaces move across each other. This occurs, typically, when a patient tries to push himself up the bed, or when a patient like Mr Salisbury is unable to move himself and a handling manoeuvre is poorly managed. The skin of the buttocks rubs against the bottom sheet and friction will result (Pendleton, 1998).

> **NB:** Patients with pressure sores cost the NHS more than £250 million each year (Arblaster, 1998). Significantly, there is also a personal accounting to be made, in terms of pain, discomfort, reduced quality of life and potential threat to life.
> (Davies et al, 1991)

2. *Pressure*: Adequate blood flow to the cells, bringing oxygen and nutrients and removing waste products, is essential for cell viability. Blood capillaries form a fragile network, allowing diffusion to take place across the cell walls. Any disruption or interference with this process means that the cells will die and thus prompt tissue breakdown and pressure sore formation.

    Capillaries are supported by collagen, but in old age it is recognised that collagen is deficient, thus affecting pressure forces. If pressure is exerted on capillaries, especially those in areas over bony prominences, they will collapse and blood flow will cease (Bridel, 1993). If pressure is spread over a large area or is of short duration, it is less likely to disrupt the blood supply so that pressure sores are less likely to develop.

3. *Shear*: This occurs when the skin sticks to a surface, the bed sheet for example, but the soft tissues underneath move in a different direction (Lawrence, 1998). When a patient slips down a bed or chair, the forces of gravity pull the skeleton downwards, but the bed surface generates enough resistance to hold the skin of the sacrum, elbows, heels etc. in the same position. Distortion of the tissues and capillaries, disrupting the blood supply, leads to tissue necrosis This process is exacerbated by the presence of surface moisture, as in incontinence (Bryant et al, 1992).

Answer to question three:
How should the risk of Mr Salisbury developing a pressure sore have been assessed, and what steps should have been taken to prevent this from happening?

It has been stated by Hergenroeder (1992) and Waterlow (1995) that an experienced nurse can look at a patient and indicate whether they are at risk of developing pressure sores. Flanagan (1997) also emphasises the role of clinical judgement in assessing the risks of contracting a pressure sore, but she takes this one step further and stresses the importance of risk assessment tools as an adjunct to practice. The use of risk assessment scales to identify patients at greatest risk of pressure damage is essential to any preventative strategy (Timmons, 1999).

Risk assessment tools

These tools help to identify a patient's risk status by quantifying a range of factors that are recognised as predisposing towards pressure sore formation, e.g. physical and mental condition, mobility levels, loss of sensation etc., but the risk assessment tool should be carefully chosen, as no scale is 100% accurate. For example, the Waterlow Score is probably the best known, but is more appropriate for acute care patients than the Norton Score, which should be used, primarily, for elderly people in support of clinical judgement, not to replace it (Dealey, 1994).

A risk assessment that includes patient-related factors, such as those listed as follows should have been completed for Mr Salisbury on his admission to hospital:

- General condition
- Ability of patient, e.g. is he able to reposition himself, unaided?
- Weight of patient
- Preferences of patient and carers
- Environment: hospital or domestic setting
- Position patient likes to be nursed in

Mr Salisbury would have been shown to be at high risk of developing a pressure sore because of his age, weight, physical health status, incontinence and inability to move, as well as other factors (see Answer to question one, p 276), so that the necessary preventive action could have been implemented as follows.

Nutritional support

This should be in the form of an appropriate nutritional assessment, which focuses on weight, appetite, ability to cook and eat, and social conditions. Mr Salisbury is very thin for his height so the importance of adequate nutrition for wound healing should not be ignored.

NB: Protein is important for wound healing as it makes antibodies and leucocytes to fight infection. Low levels of serum albumin have been shown to be a major factor in causing pressure sores to deepen and enlarge.

(Lewis, 1996)

Skin care

The skin of a patient who is incontinent is at risk of damage associated with moisture and irritation due to urine on the skin. Mr Salisbury is at risk of skin breakdown because of his incontinence, immobility, hemiparesis and poor nutritional state. It is clear that his pressure areas deteriorated due to pressure, friction, shear, tissue hypoxia and lack of nutrients.

Immobility and handling manoeuvres

The correct method of helping Mr Salisbury move from bed to chair, toilet etc. should have been ascertained to prevent injury to both the patient and his carers. Adequate space and appropriate handling equipment should always be used. Frequent changes of position and an up-to-date bed, with a pressure-relieving mattress that has cells that deflate and inflate in turn, would provide all over pressure relief and aid blood flow.

Catheterisation

Mr Salisbury was incontinent of urine, so after 48 hours and because of his poor mobility and inability to indicate his need to micturate, he was catheterised. This would prevent urine from increasing the pH of the skin, leading to inflammation and vulnerability to friction. He was then clean and dry (Austin, 1999).

Wound healing

The necrotic wound should be rehydrated with hydrogel dressings. A vapour-permeable film dressing should then be used to maintain a moist environment. At each dressing change the wound should be irrigated with normal saline, which would encourage macrophage and mitotic activity within the wound (Dealey, 1994).

Preventative strategies, with a holistic assessment, leading to an individualised care plan, would be the key processes in preventing pressure sores developing and reducing Mr Salisbury's long hospitalisation.

References

Arblaster, G. (1998). Pressure sore incidence: a strategy for reduction. Nursing Standard 2(28): 49–54.

Austin, G. (1999). Eating into resources. Nursing Times 95(11): 64–67.

Bridel, J. (1993). The aetiology of pressure sores. Journal of Wound Care 2(4): 230–238.

Bryant, R.A., Shannon, M.L., Pieper, B. (1992). Pressure ulcers. In: Bryant, R.A. (Ed.) Acute and Chronic Wounds. Nursing Management. St Louis: Mosby Year Book.

Courtenay, M. (1998) Preparations for skin conditions. Nursing Times 94(7): 54–55.

Davies, K., Strickland, J., Laurence, V., Duncan, A.S., Rowe, J. (1991). The hidden mortality from pressure sores. Journal of Tissue Viability 1: 18.

Dealey, C. (1994). The Care of Wounds. London: Blackwell Science.

Flanagan, M. (1997). Choosing pressure sore risk assessment tools. Professional Nurse 12(6): (Suppl): 3–7.

Hergenroeder, P. (1992). Pressure ulcers risk assessment: simple or complex? Decubitus 5(7): 47–52.

Lawrence, S. (1998). Tailor-made treatment. Nursing Times 94(24): 77–78.

Lewis, B. (1996). Protein levels and the aetiology of pressure sores. Journal of Wound Care 5(10): 479–482.

Nathan, A. (1997). Products for skin problems. Pharmaceutical Journal 259(6964): 606–610.

Pendleton, S. (1998). Relieving the pressure: the important points. RCN Nursing Update: Learning Unit 081. Nursing Standard 12(36): 4–18.

Timmons, J. (1999). Pressure releases. Nursing Times Nursing Homes 1(2): 26–28.

Waterlow, J. (1995). Recording risk factors. Nursing Times 91(11): 64–65.

Restraint: wandering

Vivienne Mathews

Barry Braid lives in the Maple Leaf Nursing Home. He is 91 years old and enjoys the company of other people, chatting for hours to anyone willing to listen to him tell about his childhood and his experiences during the war. Two of his greatest pleasures are to show others his album of photographs, which he carries with him at all times, and to play the piano. He sometimes sings as well.

Mr Braid appears to need little sleep and is often awake, late at night, listening to music on his radio, which; because of his increasing deafness, is very loud. He also suffers from mild dementia.

Other residents of the home are accustomed to his ways and used to enjoy a chat with him; one neighbour often left the door of her room open for Mr Braid to pop in for a cup of tea and a chat whenever he felt like it.

Recently, however, Mr Braid has been 'popping in' more and more frequently and has become a bit of a nuisance, as he calls on his neighbours at unsociable times, usually in the early hours of the morning.

One day, during a particularly long, loud session at the piano, Mr Braid was asked to stop playing. He did, but then wandered about the home, turning up, when least expected, in the kitchen, bathrooms and private rooms of other residents.

Question one: Why is 'wandering' a problem in people with dementia?
10 minutes

Question two: What information will the nursing home staff need in order to have a better understanding of elderly people with wandering tendencies?
10 minutes

Question three: What strategies can be adopted in the management of Mr Braid's wandering?
10 minutes

Time allowance: **30 minutes**

Answer to question one:
Why is 'wandering' a problem in people with dementia?

Wandering, as defined by Thomas (1995) is a purposeful behaviour that tries to fulfil a particular necessity in an individual. It is characterised by an extraordinary amount of movement that may lead to safety and/or nuisance-related problems. It has been viewed, primarily, as an uncooperative behaviour and as such, poses many problems for caregivers.

The chief fears are that the individual may become lost, may endanger other people, or be at risk of injury or death to themselves (Melillo & Futrell, 1998). These symptoms of dementia are poorly tolerated by others.

Pacing and wandering

Types

- Aimless and excessive ambulation
- Continuous searching for unattainable objects
- Night walking
- Pacing back and forth
- Exit seeking
- Trespassing.

Possible consequences

- Fatigue
- Falls
- Getting lost
- Bothering other people
- Interfering with others' belongings.

Related issues

- Agitation, followed by ambulation
- Wandering accompanied by touching, fondling, moving objects, repetitive mannerisms, throwing/handling things inappropriately, strange noises, requests for attention, uncooperative behaviour.

(Adapted from Melillo & Futrell, 1998)

Answer to question two:
What information will the nursing home staff need in order to have a better understanding of elderly people with wandering tendencies?

Based on recent findings from clinical and research literature, Cohen-Mansfield, Werner, Culpepper, Barkley (1997) found that the content of an education pro-gramme for carers could cover the following areas:

- Characteristics and causes of dementia
- Problem behaviours, e.g. wandering
- General guidelines for dealing with elderly people suffering from dementia
- Different types of pacing/wandering and their consequences
- Management strategies for dealing with this behaviour

Importantly, it should be remembered that pacing/wandering behaviour is not all bad, and may, in fact, be beneficial as it provides exercise and physical stimulation in an institutionalised elderly person.

Wandering should be accommodated as much as possible, and nursing home staff should be encouraged to apply their new knowledge to day-to-day situations. For example, what causes the wandering experienced by Mr Braid? Perhaps he had a job that involved helping people or he could have been involved with fellow workers on an intimate basis and now misses the contact he had with his colleagues. Scenarios like the one offered earlier bring to life issues that both nurses and elderly people encounter in nursing home and hospital settings. Group discussions will facilitate problem identification and possible solutions, making the transition from theory to putting new concepts into practice (Roberto, Wacker, Jewell, Rickard, 1997).

Answer to question three:
What strategies can be adopted in the management of Mr Braid's wandering?

Management strategies

Residents in general

- Try to understand the residents' needs
- Establish when, where and why the behaviour occurs
- Be flexible with providing personal care
- Maintain a calm environment
- Avoid physical restraints (may cause serious injury)
- Avoid chemical restraints (may cause serious side-effects)
- Use short, concise words and sentences
- Do not shout or lose your temper
- Use non-verbal cues.

Specifically for pacing/wandering residents

- Do not attempt to prevent or stop the behaviour (unless the environment is unsafe)
- Allow wandering in a safe place, e.g. in the corridor or in a sheltered, secure garden
- Avoid crowded areas, e.g. the kitchen
- Observe the behaviour pattern and try to accommodate the resident (the resident may be trying to find the bathroom)
- Engage the resident in conversation during wandering behaviour (distraction)
- Find an appropriate time for doing the objectionable behaviour, i.e. playing the piano
- Encourage other residents to sing along with Mr Braid
- Set parameters, e.g. only 'pop in' to neighbours, once a day, at 10.30 a.m. or 3.00 p.m.
- Find time to talk to Mr Braid and listen to him as he recounts his past.

Use if necessary

- Colour-coded identity bracelet
- Alarm-triggering bracelet
- Pictures of the resident given to receptionists near doors and exits
- Electronic locks or swipe cards for staff to activate
- Baffle locks.

(Adapted from Cohen-Mansfield et al, 1997)

References

Cohen-Mansfield, J., Werner, P., Culpepper, W.J., Barkley, D. (1997). Dementia and wandering: evaluation of an inservice training programme. Journal of Gerontological Nursing 23(10): 40–47.

Melillo, K.D., Futrell, M. (1998). Clinical outlook. Wandering and technology devices. Journal of Gerontological Nursing 24(8): 32–38.

Roberto, K.A., Wacker, R., Jewell, E.M., Rickard, M. (1997). Residents rights: knowledge and implementation by nursing staff in long term care facilities. Journal of Gerontological Nursing 23(12): 32–40.

Thomas, D.W. (1995). Wandering: A proposed definition. Journal of Gerontological Nursing 21(9): 35–41.

Further reading

Wynne-Harley, D. (1997). Living Dangerously: Risk Taking, Safety and Old People. London: Centre for the Policy on Ageing.

For Captain McDavid, it must be assumed that he planned for his retirement: had made adequate financial provision for himself, had bought an appropriate living space, was in good health and had good family contacts.

Many people dread retirement with its enforced leisure time, financial hardship, potential for boredom, changed relationships and loss of social outlets; but increasingly, there is a large body of physically active, leisure-orientated, well-educated people with wider expectations of retirement than ever before, who view retirement with a great deal of satisfaction. It may appear that Captain McDavid is amongst the latter group, accepting retirement but finding the transition between work and retirement onerous and demanding.

Answer to question three:
With reference to the theory of Disengagement, describe how Captain McDavid could be influenced to adopt a more positive attitude to retirement.

The Disengagement theory, as described by Cumming & Henry in 1961, suggests that both society and the elderly person benefit if there is a gradual, but mutual, withdrawal from each other. It maintains that the ageing process is inevitable and natural so that the individual 'disengages' from principal positions or tasks. Society then reciprocates by replacing these offices with younger members of society. The main flaw in this theory appears to be that no benefit is accrued for the elderly person, only the young who are 'upwardly mobile' (Marr & Kershaw, 1998).

This theory, stereotypically, sees elderly people as passive, tired and willing to accept a docile, compliant role. This may be true for some elderly people, but not all.

It is not known if Captain McDavid wanted to retire, to relinquish responsibility and take up cooking. If given no choice and disengagement became compulsory, or involuntary, there may not be a plan for the future, adequate financial provision or a social network to support him during this transition. Even if he had planned for his future in advance of his retirement, he could not have predicted how things would have turned out for him.

Some coping mechanisms for Captain McDavid may be to:

- Find a new role with a voluntary body, e.g. sea scouts
- Discover a fitness regimen that may provide new friends and be a positive health gain
- Discover new ways of tackling problems, as physical strength diminishes
- Find tasks that lead to meaningful goals; not playing bingo, but perhaps learning to play a musical instrument. This may lead to relationships with other musicians or joining an orchestra
- Be encouraged to take control of his life; refuse to be stereotyped as retired or leisured (Grimley-Evans, 1994)
- Develop his family contacts by keeping in touch with his nephews and their families.

Retirement can be seen by Captain McDavid as an opportunity to achieve things that his working life had prevented, consequently he may avoid activities that remind him of his former work.

Depression and despair can be the outcome of retirement, whether sought after or mandatory, as disillusionment and inertia takes hold. Captain McDavid needs to restructure his life, taking into account his age, gender, class, education and future aspirations. He may be feeling that society has let him down, but a rapidly changing environment, in technology, for example, and his own gradual decline in physical health as age advances, needs coping strategies and adaptations that can raise his self-esteem, preserve his physical abilities and reactivate his zest for life (Marr & Kershaw, 1998).

References

Cumming, E., Henry, H. (1961). Growing Old: The Process of Disengagement. New York: Basic Books.

Eliopoulos, C. (1990). Caring for the Elderly in Diverse Settings. Pennsylvania: J.B. Lippincott Company.

Farrell, J. (1990). Nursing Care of the Older Person. Pennsylvania: J.B. Lippincott Company.

Fennell, G., Phillipson, C., Evers, H. (1988). The Sociology of Old Age. England: Open University Press.

Grimley-Evans, J. (1994). Can we live to be a healthy hundred? Medical Research Council News, 64. Autumn.

Marr, J., Kershaw, B. (1998). Caring for Older People: Developing Specialist Practice. London: Arnold.

Victor, C. (1987). Old Age in Modern Society. London: Croom Helm.

Walker, A. (1991). The social construction of dependency in old age. In: Loney, M., Bocock, R., Clarke, J., Cochrane, A., Graham, P., Wilson, M. (Eds) The State or The Market. (41–55). London: Sage Publications.

Windmill, V. (1990). Ageing Today. London: Edward Arnold.

Wright, S. G. (1988). Nursing Older People. Pennsylvania: J.B. Lippincott Company.

Further reading

Gibson, H.B. (1992). The Emotional and Sexual Lives of Elderly People. London: Chapman & Hall.

Rheumatoid arthritis

Vivienne Mathews

Eliza Cooper is a 38-year-old librarian, who lives alone in a small terraced cottage on the outskirts of an historic village. She is fiercely independent, doing her own home decorating, car maintenance and household repairs.

Her only relative, a sister who is divorced with three children, lives many miles away and does not drive, so that the onus to keep in touch is on Eliza. She has few interests outside her home, preferring to stay in her garden, read or play the piano.

She noticed that for several months, she was very stiff in the mornings and that her wrists and ankles were painful and slightly swollen. After an hour or so the stiffness disappeared, but pain in her hands and feet worsened as the day progressed. She also complained of feeling very tired.

After visiting her GP, she was admitted to hospital for investigations of suspected rheumatoid arthritis.

Question one: What are the pathophysiology, signs and symptoms of rheumatoid arthritis?

15 minutes

Question two: Describe a treatment programme for Miss Cooper that will enable her to retain her independence.

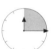

15 minutes

Question three: Discuss the major drugs used in the treatment of rheumatoid arthritis and describe their side-effects.

15 minutes

Time allowance: **45 minutes**

Answer to question one:
What are the pathophysiology, signs and symptoms of rheumatoid arthritis?

Rheumatoid arthritis occurs mostly in females, aged between 20 and 40, but can occur at any age (Hogstel, 1992). No one knows what causes the disease but a number of factors are known to trigger it: viral or bacterial infection, for example. There may be a genetic link that gives a person the potential to contract the disease.

Rheumatoid arthritis affects different people in different ways. Occasionally one or two joints are involved, but in other cases the disease is systemic, affecting every joint in the body.

About 30% of people who contract rheumatoid arthritis appear to recover completely within a few years; however about 65% of sufferers continue to have joint pain, swellings and sudden flare-ups, and about 5% become severely affected and extensively disabled (Rodwell, 1994).

It has been described as a chronic disease of the body's connective tissue that is subjected to inflammatory changes (Hogstel, 1992).

The causes of rheumatoid arthritis include:

- Idiopathic factors
- Infection
- Autoimmunity
- Metabolic abnormalities
- Genetic factors
- Psycho-social factors, e.g. stress.

(Adapted from Buckley, 1997)

According to Hogstel (1992), rheumatoid arthritis develops in four stages:

1. Synovitis: Joint inflammation (synovitis) develops, which leads to an increase in synovial fluid and thickening of the synovial membrane.
2. Pannus formation: Granulation tissue (pannus), originating from the synovial membrane, forms, extends over and destroys the articular cartilage. The joint capsule is destroyed.
3. Fibrous ankylosis: Tough, fibrous tissue replaces the pannus, thereby filling the joint space and makes movement painful.
4. Bony ankylosis: The fibrous tissue calcifies and changes the structure of the bone. The result is total immobilisation of the joint.

In this way the joints become swollen because of the increased blood flow and oedema associated with the inflammatory process. The normally sleek synovial membrane becomes thickened with fibroblasts, and inflammatory cells such as lymphocytes accumulate, which results in warm, tender, swollen joints (Voyce, 1998). The joint deformities that are characteristic of rheumatoid arthritis are the result of enzyme damage to bone and cartilage, which steadily erodes the joints. The chronic swelling of the joint makes ligaments lax and very weak, so that an unstable joint is the result (Christiansen & Grzybowski, 1993).

Answer to question two:
Describe a treatment programme for Miss Cooper that will enable her to retain her independence.

Badley (1995) states that the impact of rheumatoid arthritis on a person who lives alone is devastating. First, because of their few social contacts and then, if this is coupled with a low educational level, their problem-solving capabilities will be reduced and so their coping abilities will be severely compromised.

The major goals of treatment are to relieve pain, control symptoms, maintain mobility and preserve function in the joints – all of which will allow Miss Cooper to lead a life that is compatible with her former lifestyle (Hogstel, 1992).

The multidisciplinary health care team consisting of the rheumatology specialist nurse, nurses, occupational therapists, physiotherapists, pharmacists, dieticians, social workers, chiropodists and GPs will link together to assess and adjust care as the disease progresses (Voyce, 1998).

Drugs will be the first line of defence and are discussed in the answer to question three, but the following must also be emphasised:

- A balanced diet
- The value of rest, especially during an exacerbation of the condition
- The use of splints
- Correct posture and regular exercise, always stopping before tiredness becomes a problem
- Correct limb positioning in order to prevent deformities.

(Hill, 1995)

Obesity is to be prevented, as additional weight will increase the strain on the joints. 'Fad diets' and miracle cures should be avoided as they give false hope and are usually very expensive.

Miss Cooper should be advised not to lift anything heavy, to rest at least twice a day, to avoid fatigue, and lastly, to get a good night's sleep. Throughout the day, Miss Cooper should avoid rushing and prioritise her daily chores and activities, only doing what is strictly necessary. Relaxation, with a warm bath in the mornings to help alleviate morning stiffness and some form of mental distraction, such as hobbies and social activities, may help to relieve pain and tension (Voyce, 1998).

Answer to question three:
Discuss the major drugs used in the treatment of rheumatoid arthritis and describe their side-effects.

Control of the inflammatory process and of pain are the priorities of drug treatment in rheumatoid arthritis.

Starting with simple analgesics, such as paracetamol or co-proxamol, which have both anti-inflammatory and analgesic effects, these drugs, their dose and timing should be adjusted with each exacerbation or remission of the disease. Analgesic drugs can be bought over-the-counter without prescription, but only doctors can prescribe slightly stronger drugs, such as dextropropoxyphene. Very strong, addictive drugs, such as pethidine or morphine, are hardly ever used. A mixture of small doses of two or three different analgesics may work better than one on its own, but whatever drug is used for Eliza, she should be advised to limit its use to times when the pain is very bad, or to take it before doing something known to be painful. Severe rheumatoid arthritis may require regular analgesics to control pain and allow movement.

As the condition progresses, non-steroidal anti-inflammatory drugs (NSAIDs), such as ibuprofen, naproxen or piroxicam, should be given. As these drugs reduce inflammation, they also reduce pain, swelling and stiffness, and may, therefore, be better at relieving pain than ordinary analgesics (Rodwell, 1994). This group of drugs should be taken with food and may give rise to headaches, dizziness and gastrointestinal irritation. Eliza should be advised to take NSAIDs with or immediately after food and never on an empty stomach. She should report to her GP any gastric pain, such as indigestion and if she experiences stomach pains, a doctor should be consulted, immediately (Rodwell, 1994). Eliza should also observe the colour of her faeces as black faeces may be indicative of gastric bleeding. NSAIDs do not cure rheumatoid arthritis, but will alleviate the worst of the pain and inflammation (Badley, 1995).

A cautionary view from Voyce (1998) claims that after taking NSAIDs for 6–8 weeks, rheumatoid arthritis may increase in severity, which may mean that powerful drugs, such as methotrexate or sulphasalazine, are then used. These disease-modifying drugs (DMARDs) hinder the rate and progress of disease activity. Their effect will not be noted for 3–6 months after starting therapy, and must be monitored carefully as blood discrasias, renal and hepatic damage, dermatitis, mouth ulcers and corneal deposits may occur.

Steroids are hormones that occur naturally in the body and are used in rheumatoid arthritis to reduce inflammation and damp down the body's defence mechanisms. They can be given in tablet form or by injection into a joint that is particularly painful or given by i.m. or i.v. injection (pulse therapy) (Rodwell, 1994). They will reduce inflammation and restore joint function. Prednisolone, a corticosteroid, is often used until DMARDs begin to take effect, usually for about 8 weeks.

Some cytotoxic drugs, cyclosporin for example, and methotrexate, can be used in conjunction with DMARDs to treat chronic rheumatoid arthritis that is unresponsive to other treatment. Skin rashes, gastrointestinal ulceration and bone marrow depression are common side-effects.

It is important to be aware of the side-effects of even the most commonly used drugs, such as aspirin, as side-effects of gastric irritation, tinnitus and hearing loss may follow. All these drugs have harmful effects (Holman & Lori, 1997).

Gold injections have been used since the 1920s in the treatment of rheumatoid arthritis; this can now be taken in tablet form.

D-penicillamine can be used for people who are allergic to penicillin. A small initial dose is given, building up to a therapeutic dose over a period of several months.

Miss Cooper will have a wide range of drugs to contend with as her condition progresses. It is important for her to use them carefully, following instructions and keeping a record of how the drugs are affecting her. She should be under the supervision of her GP and the rheumatoid specialist nurse.

References

Badley, E. (1995). The impact of disabling arthritis. Arthritis Care and Research 8(4): 221–228.

Buckley, C.D. (1997). Treatment of rheumatoid arthritis. British Medical Journal 345: 236–238.

Christiansen, J.L., Grzybowski, J.M. (1993). Biology of Ageing. St Louis, MO: Mosby Year Book.

Hill, J. (1995). Patient education in rheumatic diseases. Nursing Standard 9(25): 25–28.

Hogstel, M.O. (1992). Clinical Manual of Gerontological Nursing. St Louis, MO: Mosby Year Book.

Holman, H., Lori, K. (1997). Patient education to good health care for patients with chronic arthritis. Arthritis and Rheumatism 40(8): 1371–1373.

Rodwell, L. (1994). Arthritis and Rheumatism. London: Ward Lock.

Voyce, M.A. (1998). Rheumatoid arthritis. Professional Nurse 13(7): 441–445.

Further reading

Burke, M.M., Walsh, M.B. (1992). Gerontological Nursing. St Louis, MO: Mosby Year Book.

Scabies: ageing skin changes

Vivienne Mathews

Jim and Hilda Bletchley, aged 78 and 77 respectively, live in a retirement flat that has been converted from a large mansion house, in the centre of a south coast seaside resort. They moved there from Nottingham 8 years ago, as they had always promised each other that they would retire to the coast, where they had spent many happy holidays when their children were young. They have known each other since their school days and have only spent time apart when war duties intervened.

Hilda has had rheumatoid arthritis for many years. It has now run its course, leaving Hilda with characteristic deformities: no muscle strength (she is almost immobile) and fragile, paper thin skin caused by years of steroid use.

Jim, who is the fitter of the two, has recently suffered from bronchitis and angina, both of which have left him feeling tired and irritable, and very worried about their future together.

Jim and Hilda have no children and no close relatives, but rely heavily upon their GP for advice and support. The GP thought that a stay in a rest home, together, might give Jim a break from caring for his wife, giving him the chance to rest and recuperate before winter started and his bronchitis returned. Both Jim and Hilda welcomed the idea. It would afford them a change of scenery, give new insights on how to help Hilda and give Jim a much needed break.

Whilst they were there, an outbreak of scabies was detected. Jim and Hilda were not treated for this, but on their return home started to itch and scratch their arms and hands. The doctor diagnosed scabies.

Question one: What is scabies and what are the main symptoms?
10 minutes

Question two: Outline the treatment for scabies.
10 minutes

Question three: List the changes in skin structure that occur in old age.
10 minutes

Time allowance: **30 minutes**

Client profiles in nursing: adults & the elderly

Answer to question one:
What is scabies and what are the main symptoms?

Scabies is a skin infection caused by the mite *Sarcoptes scabiei*. Scabies is an allergic reaction to this mite, which burrows into the skin to lay eggs.

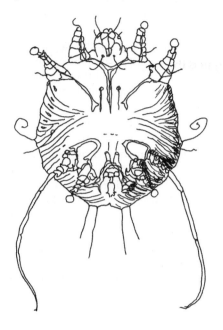

Figure 45.1: Scabies male mite.

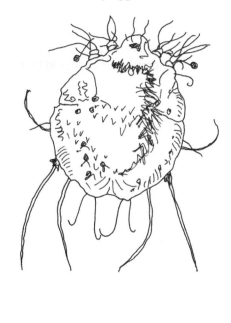

Figure 45.2: Scabies female mite.

The burrow is a thin, grey line, 1 cm long, with a small vesicle at one end containing a tiny speck, which is the mite.

It appears that the prevalence of the disease is cyclical, with a peak occurrence every 15–20 years that may last for 2–3 years before lessening in severity (Effectiveness Matters, 1999). This rise and fall has been attributed to health care workers treating cases only when the incidence reaches high levels (Green, 1989).

There is a variable incubation period, lasting from several days to about 6 weeks after contact with an infected person. Scabies is transmitted by skin-to-skin contact, in a warm environment (which would be typical of a rest home), for example by holding hands, being in bed together or sexual intimacy. A contact time of as little as 2 minutes is sufficient for infestation to occur. Scabies cannot be picked up from bed clothes or clothing, as the scabies mite cannot live long outside the human body. It cannot jump from person to person (Effectiveness Matters, 1999).

The symptoms of scabies infestation include:

● Itching: worse after a hot bath or a warm bed
● Rash: on wrists, finger webs, toes, between thighs, on trunk, round waist, axillary areas, under breasts, round nipples, penis, scrotum and buttocks.

Sexuality

Vivienne Mathews

> Noel and Judith Witt have been married for 53 years, having celebrated their Golden Wedding anniversary in 1997. They have two children, Roger and Rosalie, who are both married with children of their own.
>
> Noel is a retired civil servant and a very talented artist. Judith is a retired art teacher who taught in private schools and has had several pictures exhibited in some of the smaller London art galleries.
>
> Judith, although older than her husband, has few health problems, but recently has developed irritation in her lower limbs and, as a result of this, has a small venous ulcer on the left medial maleolus.
>
> Noel has been diagnosed as having Parkinson's disease, which has affected his ability to hold a paint brush. Noel and Judith have had an active sex life, which continues to the present time, but has now become a problem for Judith.
>
> She is 86 years old and quite happily states that sex three times a week has kept them both fit and happy.
>
> Noel had told her when she was young and naive, that if he didn't have regular sex (he meant every other day!) he would 'swell up and burst, down there!' as the sight of his erect penis proved. She still believes this to be true, but has begun to find sex unpleasant and uncomfortable.
>
> Noel is 82 and is completely unaware that his wife is experiencing any difficulty during sex. He admits to taking a lot longer over 'the business' these days, but does not see this as a problem.

Question one: What ageing changes take place in the reproductive system that may account for the difficulties that Mr and Mrs Witt have experienced?

10 minutes

Question two: What psychological issues need to be considered when advising Mr and Mrs Witt about their sexual activities?

10 minutes

Question three: As Mr and Mrs Witt are now living in a rest home, consider the practical aspects of this couple having a full and active sex life.

10 minutes

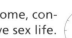

Time allowance: **30 minutes**

Answer to question one:
What ageing changes take place in the reproductive system that may account for the difficulties that Mr and Mrs Witt have experienced?

Ageing-related changes in men

- The penis becomes less sensitive than in younger men
- The rate of arousal slows considerably
- The angle of erection lowers
- The 'recovery phase' lengthens, causing the longer time span between erections
- The volume of ejaculate is reduced
- As levels of testosterone fall, the secondary male characteristics decrease: less body hair, which coarsens and greys, the voice becomes higher in pitch, breasts may develop and balding will occur (Gibson, 1992).

These changes in themselves are not a problem for Noel. It has been stated that sexual patterns remain the same throughout life (Marinaro, 1997) and as Noel has enjoyed sexual intercourse several times a week in his younger days, so he will continue to participate in sexual activities as he grows older. However, more friction is required to produce an ejaculation because of desensitisation and this has obviously become a problem for Judith.

Ageing-related changes in women

- There is less elastic tissue and more fat in the genital area
- The vulva, vagina and sometimes the breasts become less sensitive
- The vaginal mucosa becomes drier, thinner, less elastic and more fragile
- There is slower lubrication during sex. This fact alone may well account for the soreness and discomfort that Judith is experiencing during sexual intercourse (dyspareunia)
- The number of orgasms decrease
- The breasts become pendulous due to loss of adipose tissue
- Pubic hair becomes scanty
- The uterus shrinks and becomes fibrous
- There is an increased risk of infection.

(Gould, 1998)

These effects vary between individuals in the extent of their influence on sexuality, but the consequences of these ageing changes, particularly the drier, more delicate vaginal canal, will make penile penetration difficult. A satisfying continuation of sexual affection, including full intercourse, should still be attainable for Noel and Judith if this is the wish of both parties (Eliopoulos, 1990).

NB: If there is bleeding following intercourse, investigations must be carried out to exclude malignancy.

Answer to question two:
What psychological issues need to be considered when advising Mr and Mrs Witt about their sexual activities?

In the Victorian era, men and women had contradictory attitudes towards sex; whilst women were seen as having little or no sex drive and were told to endure sex in order to have children, men were said to have uncontrollable sex drives and were advised to seek out prostitutes to satisfy their carnal appetites.

Perhaps this legacy still lingers today, and yet at about the age of 60 years, seven out of 10 couples are still sexually active; at 75 years of age one out of four healthy couples remain sexually active (Gibson, 1992). In the light of these facts, health professionals should not be surprised that Noel and Judith have regular sexual intercourse.

Factors that can affect sexual activity in later life include:

Advantageous factors

- More leisure time, when not tired
- Large amounts of tenderness through years of companionship
- Fewer financial worries
- No family responsibilities
- No fear of pregnancy
- No need for contraception.

(Roberts, 1989)

Adverse factors

- Poor health
- Lack of partners
- Lack of privacy – especially the fear of being overheard
- 'Spoiled' body image
- Boredom – when sex becomes routine
- Fear of failure – especially in men.

(Adapted from Roberts, 1989)

Appropriate advice should be given to Noel, for instance, that his wife is experiencing difficulty, so a longer arousal time to allow lubrication of the vagina may be advantageous, or the judicious use of a lubricant, such as KY Jelly™, may go some way to dispel the discomfort. Perhaps Judith is caught in a vicious circle of pain, poor relaxation, more pain, and needs to feel wanted and loved in order to relax and enjoy sexual relations with her husband.

Sadly, society views the sexual habits of elderly people in a negative way, which may inhibit their expressions of sexuality (Marinaro, 1997). They are not seen as sexually desirable and interested in sex, but as 'virile at 16 and lecherous at 60!'

Answer to question three:
As Mr and Mrs Witt are now living in a rest home, consider the practical aspects of this couple having a full and active sex life.

Institutionalisation does not offer many opportunities for intimacy and/or sexuality, but if a resident's sexual concerns are discussed by non-judgemental, respectful, listening staff it will not cause uneasiness or disquiet. Sexuality, as seen written in care plans, by nurses, is an indication of their attitudes towards sex and the elderly, e.g. has own teeth, likes nails to be polished, or even, not applicable (Evans, 1999). It is important that staff in a home think of Noel's and Judith's sexual behaviour as an unmet need they try to express, rather than it being a 'problem', so that they are given the opportunity to express their sexual feelings in private.

When issuing guidelines for staff about sex and sexuality, it is vital to stress that respect for other people's sexual attitudes must be forthcoming, even when they differ from their own.

Specific interventions for sexual relations

Staff and residents would benefit from some education on topics related to sexuality; this could include:

- A supportive, private environment, with a door that has a working lock, should be provided. A 'Do not disturb' sign may be of value here. Current guidelines for rest homes ensure that all rooms can be locked by residents
- Instruction to knock on the door and wait for permission to enter
- Telling staff not to watch or evesdrop on residents' sexual activities
- Recognise the increased need amongst elderly people for touch
- Encourage alternate forms of sexual expression, such as kissing and hugging
- Provide sexual information and counsel to interested residents.
(Richardson & Lazur, 1995)

Promoting sexuality in elderly people provides them with the opportunities to live the remainder of their lives in the joy of each other's company and the warmth of an ongoing, loving relationship.

References

Eliopoulos, C. (1990). Caring for the Elderly in Diverse Settings. Pennsylvania: J.B. Lippincott Company.

Evans, G. (1999). Sexuality in old age: why it must not be ignored by nurses. Nursing Times 95(21): 46–47.

Gibson, H.B. (1992). The Emotional and Sexual Lives of Older People. London: Chapman & Hall.

Gould, D. (1998). The Menopause: sexually related problems. Royal College of Nursing: Continuing Education. Nursing Standard 12(25): 49–56.

Marinaro, D. (1997). In your turn: what do you identify as problems with sexuality for patients, families and staff in nursing homes and long term facilities? What type of interventions have you found useful. Journal of Gerontological Nursing 23(10): 52–55.

Richardson, J.P., Lazur, A. (1995). Sexuality in the nursing home patient. American Family Physician 51(1): 121–124.

Roberts, A. (1989). Sexuality in later life. Senior systems. 37. Systems of life No. 172. Nursing Times 85(24): 65–68.

Shingles

Vivienne Mathews

> Greta Travenna is a 78-year-old widow, who lives alone in a large semi-detached, double-fronted house, in a socially decaying suburb of a large south coast city. She is of German origin, having arrived in England at the start of World War II, aged 18. Greta married an Englishman, Richard Travenna, but the relationship did not last as Greta had a dictatorial nature; she was never wrong and refused, point blank, to compromise on any domestic issues, leaving Richard no choice but to leave her after 10 years of marriage. Greta has strong family ties with a cousin who lives in Germany, but no children and few friends. Greta is financially secure, but reluctant to spend money on her home.
>
> Her house, although warm, is dilapidated, with peeling paint work, threadbare carpets, no modern electrical household devices and a wooden draining board attached to a 'butler' type sink. Coal fires, in her living room and bedroom, are the main sources of heat.
>
> Greta developed shingles, typical of that in Ramsay–Hunt syndrome. It left her with a facial tic, a dry right eye, drooping, sensitive facial muscles, poor balance and a loss of feeling in her lips and mouth. Although she wears glasses, her sight was not affected.

Question one: Identify the causes, aetiology, epidemiology, and signs and symptoms of this condition.

15 minutes

Question two: What is the treatment and probable prognosis for Mrs Travenna?

15 minutes

Question three: What residual symptoms could affect Mrs Travenna 4 months after contracting the disease?

10 minutes

Time allowance: **40 minutes**

Answer to question one:
Identify the causes, aetiology, epidemiology, and signs and symptoms of this condition.

Shingles is a common disease characterised by inflammatory changes at a posterior root ganglion.

Figure 47.1 shows a cross-section of the spinal cord showing the posterior root ganglion (Ross & Wilson, 1996).

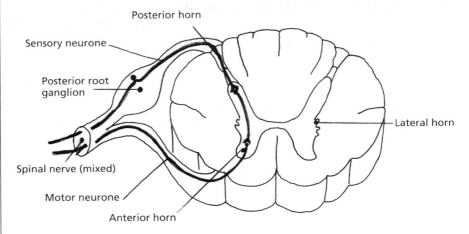

Figure 47.1: Cross-section of the spinal cord, showing posterior root ganglion.

Causes

Chicken pox (varicella) is uncomfortable in childhood but resolves within 2 or 3 weeks, leaving the causative organism – the varicella-zoster virus – ready to be reactivated in later life, particularly at times of increased stress and anxiety or ill health, when it is known as shingles (herpes zoster) (Clarke, 1998).

In old age, the normal ageing process interferes with the immune system, depressing its functions and leaving elderly people at risk of contracting shingles. In the UK, 200 000 people develop shingles each year; the incidence rises with age. The older the person who develops the condition, the more severe it tends to be, with slower recovery and more frequent and severe complications.

Both sexes are equally affected and it can occur more than once, as an attack affords only temporary immunity. It has been suggested that 1.5% of patients may experience a recurrence (MacLennan et al, 1994).

Signs and symptoms

- Malaise and fever
- Anorexia
- Burning or tingling in the area served by the affected nerve.

These symptoms may develop 2–5 days before the rash appears:

- Rash – red, maculopapular lesions
- Pain accompanying the rash
- Lesions fill with watery fluid
- Lesions taking on a pustular aspect
- Drying up and crusting of lesions
- Severe itching – may last for 3 weeks
- Crusts fall off leaving pigmented scars
- Normal pigmentation is not regained for several months
- Scarring may result if the rash is ulcerated or becomes infected.

(Adapted from Garrett, 1993)

There is intense irritation and pain. The vesicules dry up after 1–2 weeks, when itching will occur; the healing process will be longer if secondary infection is present as a result of scratching. Permanent scarring of the skin may result.

Post-herpatic neuralgia is an unpleasant sequelae that occurs particularly in elderly people. The pain is so severe and persistent that the sufferer may develop suicidal depression (Gilden, 1994).

NB: Ramsay–Hunt syndrome is a form of herpes zoster, affecting the throat and ear. Vesicular eruptions on the pinna and external auditory meatus are present, and a facial palsy of the lower motor neurone type. It is characterised by severe ear pain, facila nerve paralysis, hearing loss and vertigo.

(Houston et al, 1979)

Answer to question two:
What is the treatment and probable prognosis for Mrs Travenna?

The lesions would have to be kept clean and dry.

Regular analgesics would have to be prescribed, as well as corticosteroid therapy, which would help to lessen the pain.

Early intervention (within 48 hours of the appearance of the rash) with an antiviral agent, such as acyclovit (Zovirax), may have been effective in reducing post-herpatic neuralgia and speeding up healing (Torrens et al, 1998).

Atropine drops and antibiotic drops can be instilled into the eyes.

Idoxuridine dissolved in dimethylsulfoxide (DMSO) may be used topically – applied to the complete dermatome – for 5 days. Some elderly patients may not be able to tolerate its application, which will cause the skin to blister.

Greta should be made as physically comfortable as possible; she should be wearing loose clothes so that the rash would not be irritated. The application of lotions and ointments to the lesions, sterile dressings, cold compresses (even a bag of frozen peas would give temporary relief), relaxation and diversional therapies should be used.

Shingles would make Greta very uncomfortable; she would feel disfigured and anxious. It would be invaluable to talk to her about her anxieties (it is not a fatal disease), giving accurate information about the course of the disease and treatments that may be given. It is likely that Greta's sleep patterns would be disrupted, so that she would be feeling tired and depressed, as restless night followed restless night. A combination of analgesics and hypnotics (if pre-scribed) would therefore have been tried; comfortable positioning, with the use of bed cradles to keep heavy bed clothes off affected areas, would be seen as essential. Beverages should be given as desired and a quiet, relaxed atmosphere to reduce stress would be beneficial (Garrett, 1993).

Good nutrition, in the form of small, appetising meals and adequate fluid intake should be encouraged. Vitamin C is essential, as it would help to heal the skin eruptions by aiding the formation of collagen. Fluid balance should be monitored for signs of dyspnoea or oedema, indicating a degree of cardiovas-cular impairment common in elderly people. Post-herpatic neuralgia is some-times improved by repeated applications of an electrical vibrator over the painful area (Garrett, 1993).

Answer to question three:
What residual symptoms could affect Mrs Travenna 4 months after contracting the disease?

Mrs Travenna was an independent woman but has now become increasingly depressed and inactive. This has led to bouts of severe constipation, with poor eating habits, weight loss and accompanying lassitude.

Social isolation has become a problem as the muscles of the right side of her face have not returned to their former tension, leaving her with an acute anxiety about her physical appearance. She has a permanent dry eye, requiring artificial tears to be instilled twice a day.

Although Mrs Travenna has a hearing aid, she is not yet used to using it and so does not use it as often as she should, which increases her feelings of isolation and depression. Her balance is poor, making crossing the road, going up and down kerbs or stairs very difficult, and further compounding her isolation by an understandable reluctance to go out.

Pain or severe sensitivity in the head and face may have been treated with analgesics, but as the pain of shingles does not involve 'pain nerves' of the peripheral or central nervous system, they may have been ineffective (Caroll & Bowsher, 1993).

Referral to a pain clinic may have resulted in the decision for Mrs Travenna to have a stellate ganglion block. This involves a short stay in hospital and an injection of 15 ml plain bupivicaine 0.375% into the right side of her neck. This causes initial side-effects of a hoarse voice, a drooping right eye lid (ptosis), nasal congestion (Horner's syndrome) and transient arm weakness, but ultimately Mrs Travenna's post-herpatic neuralgia will have been alleviated with good sleeping patterns and mood enhanced by the introduction of amitriptyline (Gilden, 1994).

It will be difficult for Mrs Travenna to manage her domestic affairs, especially laying and lighting the fire, and cleaning out the ashes. Care agencies will provide carers for domestic work, such as cleaning, shopping and doing laundry, as well as giving limited personal care, in order to meet hygiene needs. Although Mrs Travenna is reluctant to spend money on herself, this intervention is vital; it not only fulfils her domestic and personal care needs, but provides social interaction at least once a day.

References

Caroll, D., Bowsher, D. (1993). Pain Management and Nursing Care. Oxford: Butterworth-Heinemann.

Clarke, K. (1998). Post herpatic neuralgia: a care study. Nursing Times 94(31): 52–53.

Garrett, G. (1993). Herpes zoster (shingles). Elderly Care 5(5): 41–46.

Gilden, D.H. (1994). Herpes zoster with post herpatic neuralgia: persisting pain and frustration. New England Journal of Medicine 330(13): 932–933.

Houston, J.C., Joiner, C.L., Trounce, J.R. (1979). A Short Textbook of Medicine. (6th ed.). London: Hodder & Stoughton.

MacLennan, W.J., Watt, B., Elder, A.T. (1994). Infections in Elderly Patients. Weston-super-Mare: Edward Arnold.

Ross, J.S., Wilson, K.J.W. (1996). Foundations of Anatomy and Physiology. London: Churchill Livingstone.

Torrens, J., Nathwani, D., MacDonald, T., Davey, P.G. (1998). Acute herpes zoster in Tayside: demographic and treatment details in immunocompetent patients, 1989–1992. Journal of Infection 36(2): 209–214.

Useful addresses

Pain Concern
PO Box 318
Canterbury
Kent CT2 0GD
Tel: 01227 710402

Shingles Support Society
41 North Road
London N7 9DP
Tel: 020 7609 9061

Stroke: dysphagia

Vivienne Mathews

Gordon Howatch is 86 years old and lives alone in a two-bedroomed, mid-terraced house on the outskirts of a small market town. He has been widowed for 8 years. He has one daughter, Daisy, who is unmarried and lives locally. She is 62 years old and works in the town's main post office as supervisor of the Complaints department. She is looking forward to her retirement in 3 years' time.

   Mr Howatch has had a chequered medical history, experiencing good health until 7 years ago, when he had a stroke. This left him with a left hemiparesis (Fig. 48.1), but with physiotherapy and a desire to 'get better', it has not been too much of a problem for him. However, last year he had another stroke, which left him with expressive dysphasia and further restricted his mobility. He was discharged from hospital 10 weeks after his stroke with a care package that consisted of the services of a home help three times a week to do shopping, light housework and meal preparation.

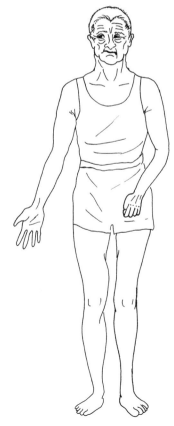

Numbness/weakness/paralysis of left side of body
Confusion, emotionalism, depression, epilepsy
Dysphasia, expressive and/or receptive
Dysarthria
Excess salivation
Homonymous hemianopia
Agnosia
Dysphagia
Shoulder subluxation
Apraxia
Disturbances of balance
Disturbances to bladder and bowel control

Figure 48.1: Effects of right hemisphere stroke and left hemiparesis.

Although designated 'self-caring' Mr Howatch had drastically reduced mobility, was unable to use the stairs, and had a wheelchair in which Daisy was able to take him out. He communicated using a picture board.

Daisy became his main carer, but because of her work commitments, was not able to help him as much as she would have liked, except at weekends. Mr Howatch was admitted to an acute elderly care ward with a 3-day history of vomiting and recent weight loss (3 kg in 2 weeks). He was diagnosed as having dysphagia.

Daisy stated that he had been increasingly unable to cope, but insisted that he wanted to remain in his own home.

Question one: What are the common physical problems and complications associated with a stroke?

15 minutes

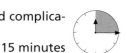

Question two: Outline the role of the multidisciplinary team, in particular the role of the speech therapist, in the treatment for dysphagia.

20 minutes

Question three: Describe the emotional problems that may be experienced by Mr Howatch and his daughter following his return home.

15 minutes

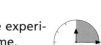

Time allowance: **50 minutes**

Answer to question one:
What are the common physical problems and complications associated with a stroke?

Incidence

Stroke is the third most frequent cause of death in the UK, after cancer and myocardial infarction (Gibbon, 1995). Stroke accounts for 10–12% of all deaths in the UK, with nearly 90% of those who subsequently die over the age of 65 (Wolfe, 1996).

One-quarter of those who die from stroke do so in the first month, but some elderly people live for many years after a stroke. Of those who do survive, one-third are not functionally independent after 1 year. Psychological sequelae are also significant, which Wolfe (1996) describes as the long-term misery of a stroke.

Predisposing factors

- Hypertension
- Smoking
- Obesity
- Heart disease
- Diabetes
- Female sex
- Hypotension
- Atheroma
- Cardiac arrhythmias
- Diet
- Alcohol consumption
- Family history of stroke.

Causes

- Cerebral thrombosis or embolism
- Cerebral haemorrhage
- Ischaemia
- Infarction.

(Adapted from Kyriazis, 1994)

Common physical problems

- Hemiplegia
- Aphasia/dysphasia (inability/difficulty in communicating)
- Aphagia/dysphagia (inability/difficulty in swallowing)
- Hemianopia (visual loss towards affected side)

- Agnosia (neglect of affected side)
- Difficulties with balance and mobility
- Incontinence.

Common psychological problems

- Memory loss (both short and long term)
- Perceptual problems
- Depression
- 'Numbness'
- Emotional lability
- Feelings of isolation
- Changes in roles
- Financial/work concerns.

Complications following a stroke

- Deep vein thrombosis (DVT)
- Urinary tract infections (UTIs)
- Pneumonia
- Pressure sores
- Contractures
- Shoulder pain/dislocations/subluxations
- Depression
- Incontinence
- Hypostatic pneumonia
- Personality changes
- Aspiration pneumonia
- Dehydration
- Urinary retention.

(Adapted from Barrett, 1992)

It may be that Mr Howatch will develop some aggressive behaviours towards Daisy, or his nurse. This displaced anger is used to relieve tension, which is almost unbearable at times (Barnett et al, 1987).

Aggressive behaviour may become apparent when Mr Howatch feels he is not getting the attention he needs. Completely unaware of other patients and how busy the nurses are, Myco (1983) identifies this self-centred aggressive behaviour as part of a stroke. It is part of the rehabilitation process. Mr Howatch is rehearsing his emotions: he is finding out, or experimenting, as to what he can expect from others in the future.

Answer to question two:
Outline the role of the multidisciplinary team, in particular the role of the speech therapist, in the treatment for dysphagia.

Dysphagia needs to be actively managed in order to ensure effective nourishment for Mr Howatch, so that he will be able to improve his chance of rehabilitation and reduce his length of stay in hospital. The care of Mr Howatch, following his stroke, requires a multidisciplinary team consisting of the patient, his family, doctors, nurses, physiotherapists, occupational therapists, speech therapists, social workers and dieticians. Other professionals who may be needed are chiropodists, dentists, hairdressers, etc.

Short, realistic goals, which involve all members of the health care team, are considered to be the most effective in helping Mr Howatch to achieve maximum independence (Gibbon, 1995).

Each member of the team has a specific contribution to make, so that an awareness of each other's roles assists with continuity of care. Failure of the multidisciplinary team will lead to fragmented care which, ultimately, will delay the rehabilitation process for Mr Howatch. Conflict and petty jealousies between the various team members are reported to have been the result of a lack of understanding of each other's roles (Gibbon, 1995).

Once goals and interventions are agreed, Daisy should be involved in her father's care, reinforcing the multidisciplinary team's teaching when at home.

Speech therapy will play a vital part in Mr Howatch's rehabilitation. Dysphagia, or difficulty in swallowing, has been identified. It has been estimated that approximately 40–60% of patients who have had a stroke will have some degree of dysphagia (Gordon, 1987).

Dysphagia, which may have developed when Mr Howatch became ill, causes drooling, coughing (before, during or after swallowing), and food pockets to be found in the mouth. He may have regurgitation and/or a 'gurgly' voice. The speech therapist will be able to offer specific advice for these conditions (Barrett, 1992).

Oral intake: appropriate stages

Food

- Smooth paste
- Smooth puree
- Soft option with extra gravy or sauce
- Soft option that may require some chewing
- Normal diet.

Textures to avoid

- Stringy
- Crumbly

- Mixed
- Bitty
- Dry
- Sticky
- Chewy
- Tough.

Fluid

- Thickened fluids
  - Restricted
  - Unrestricted
- Cold water (supervised)
  - Teaspoons, small sips
  - Restricted
  - Unrestricted
- Cold drinks
  - As above
- Warm drinks
  - As above
- Unrestricted drinks.

(Adapted from Dangerfield & Sullivan, 1999)

Points to watch

- Thin fluids run down the throat without swallowing
- Observe person constantly while eating
- Sit person up to eat or drink
- Give food in small, bite-sized pieces
- Advise person to eat slowly
- Ensure food is not too hot or too cold
- Record food input and output on food and fluid chart
- Remember that person may have difficulty in taking medication
- Check that dentures are a good fit.

(Adapted from Beadle, 1995)

NB: Dysphasia – may be receptive or expressive.

Mr Howatch, after his stroke last year, was left with expressive dysphasia. He had the inability to express his thoughts in words. When asked by the nurse 'Who am I?', it was clear that he understood the question, but was unable to articulate the word 'nurse'; instead he pointed to a table! Shaw (1991) discusses the notion that a loss of communication skills is the most frightening and frustrating feature of a stroke.

The speech therapist's input is vital when helping carers and patients to come to terms with the frustrations that lack of speech inevitably brings. They may offer the following guidelines:

- Always speak slowly and clearly
- Facing the person will help with lip reading and comprehension
- Use short sentences
- Avoid questions that require yes/no answers, as these are words that may be mixed up
- Allow time for answers
- Use an environment free of distractions, other noise in particular
- Use writing and drawing.

(Gibbon, 1995)

Answer to question three:
Describe the emotional problems that may be experienced by Mr Howatch and his daughter following his return home.

The effects of a stroke are 'unanticipated and devastating' (Nolan & Nolan, 1998). Life changes dramatically for everyone after a stroke, so that coming to terms with physical disabilities and communication problems are bad enough, but the emotional consequences of a stroke can be as hard to deal with for both parties as the physical effects:

- *Depression*: This is a common, serious complication of a stroke and is likely to have occurred after Mr Howatch's initial recovery, when he first became aware of his disabilities and their effect on his life (Smith, 1991). He may well have suffered from feelings of sadness, powerlessness and pessimism, loss of appetite and sleep problems (Health, 1996). Grieving over what has been lost – independence, dignity, earnings, self-governance, physical appearance etc. – is part of a normal coping process, so Daisy should encourage her father to express his feelings of loss, to socialise with old friends, to go out whenever possible, ask people to call and find interests that he can enjoy.
- *Outbursts*: After a stroke it is likely that Mr Howatch will have sudden outbursts of crying or laughter. No obvious reason will be found for this, as the crying and laughter does not reflect what the person is feeling, but because of changes in the brain, caused by the stroke, no control is possible over these two emotions. Tears and giggles happen against their will and is known as 'reflex crying or laughing'. It is more often apparent with a left-sided disability (Health, 1996). This condition may resolve with time, but Daisy will have to remain calm, to resist telling her father to 'stop it!' because he won't be able to, and to explain this phenomenon to friends, visitors and family.
- *Apathy*: It may be that Mr Howatch will have lost interest in his surroundings; he may sit doing nothing for hours, or be unable to show any initiative or even to look after his own basic needs.

   Daisy will find this passiveness very frustrating, but she should come to realise that it is not due to laziness or stubbornness. She may be able to encourage Mr Howatch to make decisions, e.g. have charge of the TV remote control or what clothes he wants to wear. If he is unenthusiastic about any activities, she should still go ahead and organise them and he will join in if it is a 'given' (Health, 1996).
- *Irritability*: Mr Howatch has been an even-tempered person prior to his stroke, but now appears to have a 'short fuse' and loses control over his temper because of damage to his brain, caused by the stroke. He may be reacting to frustrations about the effects of his stroke and the swearing/ranting may be an important means of communication for him. Daisy, again, may find this difficult to cope with, but should remember that outbursts of this nature are not directed towards her, personally. She should not give in to unreasonable demands made by her father.

Answer to question two:
Describe some of the methods used to manage tinnitus and the treatment available.

The GP may be able to offer reassurance that there is no serious, underlying illness and that the noises heard are real and not imaginary. He will be able to provide information and facts about tinnitus, as well as advice on coping with it. He may also be able to refer Camilla to other professionals for further help, for a hearing aid trial, for example, if tests reveal a hearing loss.

Hearing aids are used because the less Camilla hears of external sounds, the more likely she is to be aware of tinnitus-type sounds. A hearing aid should always be fitted by an audiologist (Jeffrey, 1995).

Another form of help might be to use a masker or white noise generator. A tinnitus masker provides a means of alternative sounds, which has the ability to mask other sounds, so that the patient will be less aware of their tinnitus when there is some sort of background noise. The sound often resembles a 'sushing' noise. A white noise generator can be used for varying lengths of time, which may result in reduced awareness of tinnitus-type noises.

Tinnitus can cause great psychological stress. A high level of stress or anxiety, caused by other stressors, or the tinnitus itself, will increase the likelihood that habituation (see Answer to question three, p. 334) will not occur readily. Anger, for example, makes it more likely that Camilla will be paying attention to her tinnitus for some time to come. This situation will not improve until her anger recedes or is dispersed.

Reducing tension by counselling, cognitive therapy or relaxation techniques will take time, but will be beneficial to Camilla in the long run.

- *Relaxation*: this involves learning a method of relaxation that suits the patient and so breaks the cycle of increased tension/awareness of tinnitus/increased tension
- *Cognitive therapy*: this involves changing the way a patient thinks about the condition, entailing discussions to put the disease into perspective and so causing the patient to think more positively and help themselves to learn not to respond to the noises. Referral to a psychologist is needed for this
- *Counselling*: this is less formal than cognitive therapy and can be readily available to the patient. Tinnitus needs to be talked through with someone who can explain, rationalise and understand hearing loss.

There are also several associations and self-help groups (see useful addresses after references).

Answer to question three:
How can Camilla, with her sister's help, manage her tinnitus?

More than 85% of people with tinnitus are not bothered by it because of a natural process called 'habituation', which does not allow any attention to be paid to the internal noises. People can live with this condition and are not significantly troubled by it, because they have gone through a process of deciding that a sound such as whistling, hissing, rushing or jangling has no importance and in consequence can be ignored. It can take anything from 3 months to 18 months to achieve this state.

Camilla may have an unpredictable type of tinnitus, or have a high degree of anxiety with negative feelings about it, which will hinder the process of habituation.

As Camilla has been unable to enjoy a good night's rest, she should be advised to:

- Go to bed only when she is tired
- Buy a relaxation tape or learn a relaxation technique
- Establish a pre-bed routine, e.g. with a hot milky drink or a nightcap
- Try not to think about going to sleep; try to imagine a pleasant, positive image
- Use a tape recorder and pillow speaker to mask sounds without disturbing others
- Try a blocking technique: repeat a word or sound by saying it without sound, rather than just thinking it
- Discuss sleep problems with her sister and/or the family doctor if she needs further help.

Masking techniques and distraction could be used by Camilla to help her cope with tinnitus. Masking has an external source, so can be controlled to please her mood. If this strategy works, then Camilla should use it when her tinnitus is most troublesome. The use of low-level masking noise may allow Camilla to read, relax and enjoy Coronation Street once more.

Distraction consists of partaking in activities that will absorb all her attention and so prevent her from listening to, or dwelling on, her tinnitus. She should take up a hobby or go to an evening class, for example. Camilla should be encouraged to seek out her sister and explain that she is more irritable in the evenings, because the tinnitus is harder to cope with when she is tired. They should try doing relaxation exercises together.

NB: It is a sad fact that tinnitus in an older person is 'seldom cured, but often comforted.'

(Ross et al, 1991, p. 7)

References

Jeffrey, L. (1995). Hearing Loss and Tinnitus. London: Ward Lock.

Oxford Concise Medical Dictionary (4th ed.) (1994). Oxford: Oxford University Press.

Ross, V., Echevarria, K.H., Robinson, B. (1991). Geriatric tinnitus: causes, clinical treatment and prevention. Journal of Gerontological Nursing 17(10): 6–11.

Rutishauser, S. (1994). Physiology and Anatomy: A Basis for Nursing and Health Care. London: Churchill Livingstone.

Useful addresses

British Tinnitus Association (BTA)
Room 6
14/18 West Bar Green
Sheffield S1 2DA
Tel: 01742 796600

British Deaf Association (BDA)
38 Victoria Place
Carlisle
Cumbria CA1 1HU
Tel: 01228 58844 (voice and minicom)

Hearing Aid Council
Moorgate House
201 Silbury Boulevard
Central Milton Keynes
Bucks MK4 1LZ
Tel: 01908 585442

Urinary incontinenece

Barbara Marjoram

Yvonne Whelon, aged 54, is married to Reg and has three children. Her children, aged 19, 23 and 28 have all left home; the youngest is at University and the remaining two are married with young families. She enjoys her role of grandmother and finds her job as a schoolteacher fits into childminding in the holidays, although at times feels she could do with some free time to pursue her hobby of watercolour painting.

Yvonne has been experiencing progressively worsening urinary incontinence for the past 2 years. She is extremely embarrassed by this and has tried to hide the 'problem'. She has been wearing pads but she now feels uncomfortable and 'smelly', especially when the weather is hot. Her health has generally been good and she is postmenopausal.

Yvonne has now made an appointment with her GP to seek advice.

Question one: Define incontinence and identify how it might affect Yvonne's lifestyle.

5 minutes

Question two: Identify and explain the four types of urinary incontinence, listing at least two causes of each.

5 minutes

Question three: Yvonne has been diagnosed as suffering from urge and stress urinary incontinence. What treatments might she be offered?

5 minutes

Question four: Yvonne is advised to practice pelvic floor exercises. These are primarily intended to increase the strength of which muscles? What instruction should be given to her?

5 minutes

Time allowance: **20 minutes**

Answer to question one:
Define incontinence and identify how it might affect Yvonne's lifestyle.

Incontinence can be defined as 'the involuntary loss of urine and/or faeces at an inappropriate time or in an inappropriate place' (Marjoram, 1999 in Hogston & Simpson, 1999).

It is not a disease but a symptom of an underlying disorder that can be physical, social, mental or environmental.

Cheater (1995) identified that 'incontinence can have an adverse physical, psychological, social and economic consequence for the sufferer, family and carers'. Yvonne may become progressively disinclined to leave the security of her home, where she is near toilet and washing facilities. She may feel the need to take time off work as her employment necessitates her being physically close to her pupils when giving them advice about their work. She may withdraw from social gatherings as she feels smelly and she may also feel 'dirty'.

Answer to question two:
Identify and explain the four types of urinary incontinence, listing at least two causes of each.

1. *Stress incontinence* is more common in females than males. On physical exertion, sneezing, coughing or laughing a small amount of urine may leak. This is caused by a weakness of the supporting pelvic floor muscles, which results in an incompetent urethral sphincter. Predisposing factors include: childbirth, hormonal changes during the menopause, obesity, constipation or vaginal prolapse.
2. *Urge incontinence* is caused by detrusor muscle instability (unstable bladder), outflow obstruction and neuropathic conditions. The individual may experience the loss of a variable amount of urine with little or no warning. The cause of urge incontinence may include urinary tract infection (UTI), urethral stricture, faecal impaction, Alzheimer's disease, cerebrovascular accident and spinal cord lesions. Individuals often experience both urge and stress incontinence – especially in the elderly.
3. *Reflex incontinence* is caused by damage to the peripheral nerves to the bladder or spinal cord. The individual fails to recognise the need to micturate, causing the bladder to fill and empty on a reflex cycle. Reflex incontinence is often combined with incomplete voiding and a high residual urine volume.
4. *Overflow incontinence* is caused by urinary retention with overflow. This may be caused by obstruction from urethral stricture or faecal impaction, hypotonic bladder caused by neuropathy and anticholinergic medication or detrusor–sphincter dysynergia (uncoordinated muscle activity); this is caused by neuropathic conditions, for example multiple sclerosis and paraplegia (Marjoram, 1999 in Hogston & Simpson, 1999).

Answer to question three:
Yvonne has been diagnosed as suffering from urge and stress urinary incontinence. What treatments might she be offered?

Yvonne may be advised to do pelvic floor exercises, insert weighted cones into her vagina for varied periods of time and as she is postmenopausal, she may be prescribed hormone replacement therapy (Pomfret, 1993). Due to her post-menopausal status, Yvonne will have a decrease in the hormone oestrogen, which causes atrophic (loss of firmness in the tissue) changes in her vagina and around her urethra. This may result in inflammation which can cause urge and stress urinary incontinence symptoms (see Useful Website).

Answer to question four:
Yvonne is advised to practice pelvic floor exercises. These are primarily intended to increase the strength of which muscles? What instruction should be given to her?

Pelvic floor exercises are primarily intended to increase the strength of the levator ani muscles. Yvonne will be required to contract and relax the muscles that surround the vagina and anus, therefore improving their tone. To do this, Yvonne should be advised to either stand, sit or lie in a comfortable position while tightening the pelvic floor muscles for approximately 10 seconds and repeating this 10 times. She should experience a feeling of tightening around the anus but not in the buttocks, abdomen or legs. This procedure should be repeated twice daily. If she experiences difficulties while learning this exercise she could insert a finger into the vagina and squeeze it (Marjoram, 1999 in Hogston & Simpson, 1999). She should be encouraged to persist with these exercises as it may take 3 months before an improvement is noticed.

References

Cheater, F. (1995). Promoting urinary continence. Nursing Standard 21 June: 9(39): 33–39.
Marjoram, B. (1999). Elimination. In: Hogston, R., Simpson, P.M. (Eds) Foundations of Nursing Practice. Basingstoke: Macmillan: pp. 154–158.
Pomfret, I.J. (1993). Stress incontinence. Practice Nursing (15): 25.

Further reading

Phillips, W. (1998). How to manage stress incontinence. Practice Nurse 16(6): 364–368.
Rose, J. (1999), Making contact. Nursing Times 95(18): 75–82.
Willis, J. (1997). Use it or lose it. Nursing Times 93(15): 70–73.

Useful Website

Access to care and treatment: causes of incontinence. http://wellweb.com/ACCT/causes3.htm (Accessed 1999, July 14)